# Quick Draw

# ANATOMY

# For Anaesthetists

# Quick Draw

# ANATOMY

# For Anaesthetists

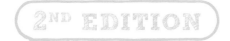

2ND EDITION

## Joanna Oram Fox

MBBCh, FRCA, FAcadMEd
Consultant Anaesthetist, Regional Anaesthesia Lead Cardiff

Scion

**© Scion Publishing Ltd, 2024**

Second edition published 2024

First edition published 2018

A CIP catalogue record for this book is available from the British Library.

ISBN 9781914961434

**Scion Publishing Limited**

The Old Hayloft, Vantage Business Park, Bloxham Road, Banbury OX16 9UX, UK

www.scionpublishing.com

**Important Note from the Publisher**

The information contained within this book was obtained by Scion Publishing Ltd from sources believed by us to be reliable. However, while every effort has been made to ensure its accuracy, no responsibility for loss or injury whatsoever occasioned to any person acting or refraining from action as a result of information contained herein can be accepted by the authors or publishers.

Readers are reminded that medicine is a constantly evolving science and while the authors and publishers have ensured that all dosages, applications and practices are based on current indications, there may be specific practices which differ between communities. You should always follow the guidelines laid down by the manufacturers of specific products and the relevant authorities in the country in which you are practising.

Although every effort has been made to ensure that all owners of copyright material have been acknowledged in this publication, we would be pleased to acknowledge in subsequent reprints or editions any omissions brought to our attention.

Registered names, trademarks, etc. used in this book, even when not marked as such, are not to be considered unprotected by law.

Artwork by Hilary Strickland

Typeset by Medlar Publishing Services Pvt Ltd, India

Printed in the UK

Last digit is the print number: 10 9 8 7 6 5 4 3 2 1

# Contents

# Preface to the first edition

I have always found anatomy a tricky subject: it was my 'last minute' subject when revising for exams. During final FRCA preparation, both I and Kiran Singh-Kandola realised that drawing simplified diagrams helped us to label any anatomy image shown to us, and so it might help others too.

This idea stayed an idea for a long time. I then started teaching some of the diagrams to core trainees studying for the primary FRCA. They seemed enthused to have an easy way to learn anatomy, but there seemed to be no revision books which did this.

I developed the step-by-step approach to drawing the diagrams from the way I taught people to draw them. In the last few years I have added many more drawings/diagrams, with the aim of covering most of the syllabus for anatomy.

Many of the diagrams are done in a step-by-step 'how to draw' method. For some topics, such as the eye and the spleen, rather than step-by-step drawing, the salient points and general anatomy needed for the exams are covered.

The main idea of the book is to make anatomy simpler for you to learn. Lots of tips are included, some about how to draw and some to help you answer some common questions. The book should aid you in all primary and final FRCA exam revision.

*Joanna Oram Fox*
*Cardiff*

# Acknowledgments

I would like to thank Kiran Singh-Kandola for being a great revision partner. From the inception of this idea, we designed simple diagrams to help us remember complicated anatomy. He was involved with the original drawings of the trigeminal nerve, cervical plexus, parts of the eye, epidural space, caudal anatomy, brachial plexus, cubital fossa, wrist, femoral canal and popliteal fossa.

# About the author

Dr Joanna Oram Fox graduated in medicine from Cardiff University in 2007. She obtained certificates of clinical excellence in medicine, surgery and general practice and won the prestigious Willie Seager surgery prize.

Joanna worked four general years as a junior doctor covering medicine, surgery, obstetrics and gynaecology, paediatrics and emergency medicine. During this time she worked in Australia and developed an interest in anaesthetics.

Joanna completed anaesthetic training in 2018 with a specialist interest in advanced airway and regional anaesthesia. She then completed a post-CCT fellowship in the Royal Perth Hospital, Australia. During her time in Perth, she worked alongside the renowned Dr Andrew Heard in the wetlab, teaching 'Can't intubate, can't oxygenate' scenarios, both in Australia and Taiwan.

On her return to the UK Joanna worked for a time in Taunton and then returned to her home hospital and Trust, Cardiff and Vale. She is currently the regional anaesthesia lead for the department.

She recently published *Quick Draw Anatomy for Medical Students*, a more comprehensive anatomy book, but based around the same simple style of illustration.

# Abbreviations

| | |
|---|---|
| AFOI | awake fibreoptic intubation |
| ASIS | anterior superior iliac spine |
| CD | collecting duct |
| CF | cubital fossa |
| CN | cranial nerve |
| DCT | distal convoluted tubule |
| EJV | external jugular vein |
| FCR | flexor carpi radialis |
| FCU | flexor carpi ulnaris |
| FO | foramen ovale |
| FR | foramen rotundum |
| FRCA | Fellow of the Royal College of Anaesthetists |
| GFR | glomerular filtration rate |
| IJV | internal jugular vein |
| IMA | inferior mesenteric artery |
| IOP | intraocular pressure |
| IVC | inferior vena cava |
| LAD | left anterior descending |
| LMS | left main stem |
| MN | median nerve |
| PCT | proximal convoluted tubule |
| PL | palmaris longus |
| RA | radial artery |
| RBC | red blood cell |
| RMS | right main stem |
| SCM | sternocleidomastoid muscle |
| SLN | superior laryngeal nerve |
| SM | somatic motor |
| SMA | superior mesenteric artery |
| SOF | superior orbital fissure |
| SPG | sphenopalatine ganglion |
| SS | somatic sensory |
| SVC | superior vena cava |
| UA | ulnar artery |
| UN | ulnar nerve |
| VS | visceral sensory |

# How to use the book

For the anatomical sections that have step-by-step drawings, the idea is to learn how to draw each diagram quickly and efficiently.

At each stage the diagram follows conventional labelling:

- Green for nerves
- Blue for veins
- Red for arteries
- Black for structures

For subsequent steps the colours are shown as tints to allow you to easily see the new lines drawn in the next step.

Once you can draw diagrams without thinking (e.g. using the shape memos like 'diamond' for the popliteal fossa), then you should learn to label them.

Finally, you should learn to explain what you are drawing. For example, the brachial plexus can be drawn in less than 15 seconds. Then you explain it whilst drawing, which should take around a minute. This will give an excellent impression in viva or OSCE examinations.

Happy drawing!

# 1.1 ▶ Circle of Willis

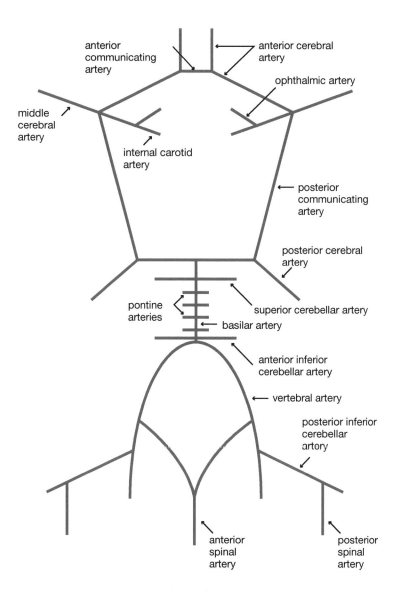

anterior communicating artery

anterior cerebral artery

ophthalmic artery

middle cerebral artery

internal carotid artery

posterior communicating artery

posterior cerebral artery

pontine arteries

superior cerebellar artery

basilar artery

anterior inferior cerebellar artery

vertebral artery

posterior inferior cerebellar artory

anterior spinal artery

posterior spinal artery

This is a notorious question that people dread. It's a complicated area to learn. However, this is the simplest diagram I could come up with that includes relevant and necessary branches. I like to think of it as an **'insect with a tail'**.

## How to draw

### STEP 1

- Draw an irregular hexagon with a small top horizontal line and a long bottom horizontal line (as shown). Draw two lines (antennae) up from the top two corners. These are the anterior cerebral arteries. The line joining them is the anterior communicating artery.

- The line going from the anterior cerebral artery to the posterior cerebral artery (see Step 3) represents the posterior communicating artery.

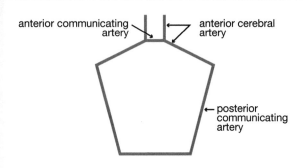

anterior communicating artery

anterior cerebral artery

posterior communicating artery

### STEP 2

- Draw 2 lines (front legs) through the second and fifth angles on the hexagon. These represent the middle cerebral artery (MCA) laterally and the internal carotid artery (ICA) medially. The ophthalmic artery branches anteriorly from the ICA.

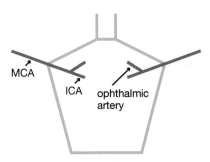

MCA

ICA    ophthalmic artery

### STEP 3

- Draw 2 lines (back legs) from the lower angles of the hexagon. These represent the posterior cerebral arteries.

- Draw 1 line from the centre of the lower, longer horizontal line on the hexagon. This represents the basilar artery.

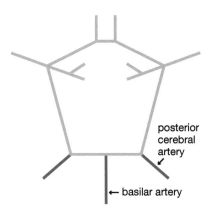

posterior cerebral artery

basilar artery

## STEP 4

Drawing 'the tail':

- Draw 6 lines horizontally through the basilar artery; the top and bottom ones should be longer than the middle ones. The top one is the superior cerebellar artery (often implicated in trigeminal neuralgia), and the bottom one is the anterior inferior cerebellar artery. The small ones represent the pontine arteries.

- Draw a downward U shape from the base of the basilar artery. These represent the vertebral arteries.

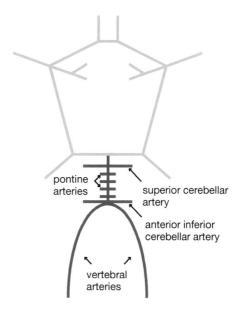

## STEP 5

- Draw horizontal lines outwards from midway along each vertebral artery. These represent the posterior inferior cerebellar arteries (PICA).

- Draw a small line from each of these to represent the posterior spinal arteries.

- Draw two curved lines, one from the inside of each vertebral artery, that join in the middle to form the anterior spinal artery.

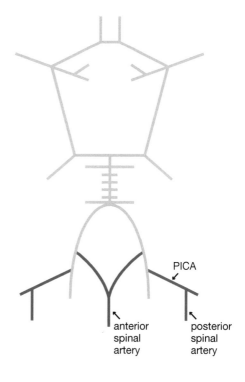

# 1.2 Venous drainage of the brain

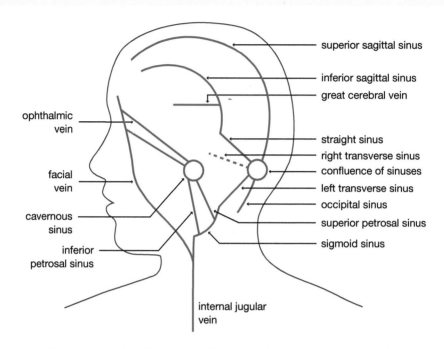

The venous drainage of the brain is often overlooked, despite the fact we have to learn the circle of Willis. It can be asked about in the FRCA. The image that I have designed is a simplified version; not every vein/sinus is included, but the important ones are.

## How to draw

### STEP 1

- Draw a head facing left. Draw the semicircle just inside the upper skull; this is the superior sagittal sinus.

- Draw a circle at the lower end of the semicircle. The circle represents the confluence of sinuses.

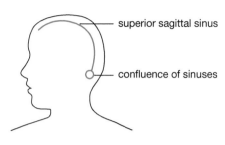

superior sagittal sinus

confluence of sinuses

### STEP 2

- From the confluence of sinuses draw a straight line heading towards just above the eye. This is the straight sinus.

- Then draw an arc curving around the eye and a line branching from this. The main arc is the inferior sagittal sinus. The branch is the great cerebral vein.

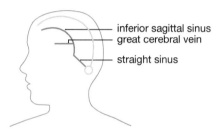

inferior sagittal sinus
great cerebral vein

straight sinus

### STEP 3

- Draw a line downwards from the confluence of sinuses; this is the occipital sinus.

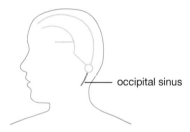

occipital sinus

### STEP 4

- Draw a line anterior to the occipital sinus as shown. This represents the left transverse sinus; it drains into the sigmoid sinus which in turn drains into the internal jugular vein (IJV).

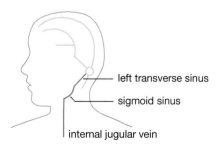

left transverse sinus

sigmoid sinus

internal jugular vein

**STEP 5**

- Draw the facial vein draining into the IJV (it does so via the common facial vein).

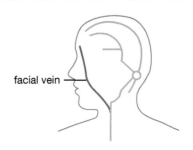

facial vein

**STEP 6**

- Draw 2 lines (the inferior and superior petrosal sinuses) upwards from the sigmoid sinus that form a blue circle (the cavernous sinus). Draw 2 lines from the facial vein to the cavernous sinus; these are the ophthalmic veins.

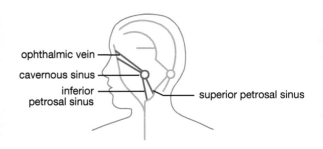

ophthalmic vein

cavernous sinus

inferior petrosal sinus

superior petrosal sinus

**STEP 7**

- Draw in a dotted line behind the left transverse sinus (to show that the line is further back). This is the right transverse sinus. Drawing all the veins on both sides would be much more complicated, but they would look similar to the left side.

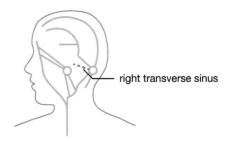

right transverse sinus

# 1.3 Venous drainage in the neck

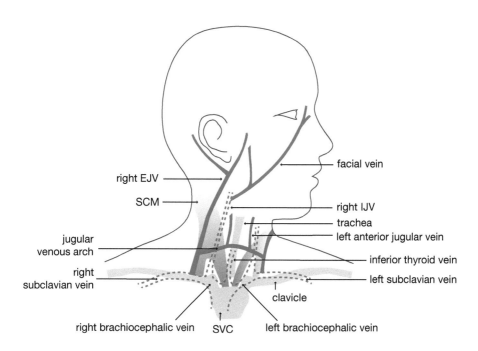

EJV   external jugular vein
IJV   internal jugular vein
SCM   sternocleidomastoid
SVC   superior vena cava

The venous drainage of the neck is the next diagram down from the venous drainage of the head.

## How to draw

### STEP 1

- Draw the head (facing right), neck, clavicles, sternum, sternocleidomastoid and trachea.

- With blue dotted lines to represent deep structures, draw the right and left internal jugular veins (IJV) draining into the brachiocephalic veins. These then meet on the right side of the body to form the superior vena cava (SVC).

- Between the 2 IJVs draw a line in front of the trachea to represent the inferior thyroid vein.

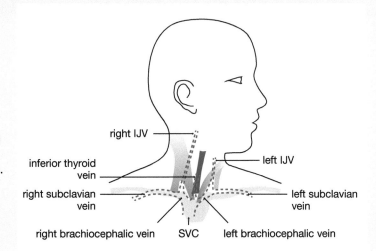

### STEP 2

- With a full blue line draw the left and right external jugular veins (EJV). These drain the external cranium and the deep parts of the face.

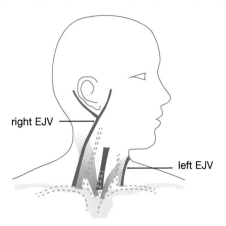

**STEP 3**

- Draw an arch that joins the 2 external jugular veins. This is the jugular venous arch. From here, draw the anterior jugular veins. There are normally two but sometimes there is only one.

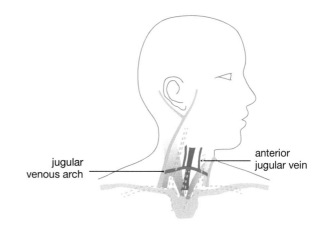

jugular venous arch

anterior jugular vein

**STEP 4**

- Draw the facial vein draining into the common facial vein which drains into the IJV.

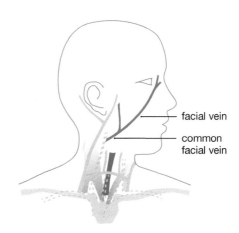

facial vein

common facial vein

# 1.4 ▸ Base of the skull

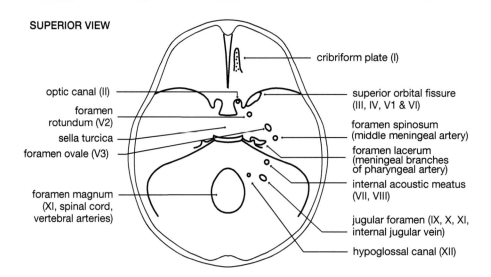

SUPERIOR VIEW

cribriform plate (I)

optic canal (II)

foramen rotundum (V2)

sella turcica

foramen ovale (V3)

superior orbital fissure (III, IV, V1 & VI)

foramen spinosum (middle meningeal artery)

foramen lacerum (meningeal branches of pharyngeal artery)

internal acoustic meatus (VII, VIII)

foramen magnum (XI, spinal cord, vertebral arteries)

jugular foramen (IX, X, XI, internal jugular vein)

hypoglossal canal (XII)

List of cranial nerves

| | | | |
|---|---|---|---|
| I | olfactory nerve | VI | abducens nerve |
| II | optic nerve | VII | facial nerve |
| III | oculomotor nerve | VIII | vestibular nerve |
| IV | trochlear nerve | IX | glossopharyngeal nerve |
| V | trigeminal nerve – | X | vagus nerve |
| | 1 ophthalmic division | XI | accessory nerve |
| | 2 maxillary division | XII | hypoglossal nerve |
| | 3 mandibular division | | |

The base of skull foramen and cranial nerve (CN) anatomy is normally asked about in the OSCE part of the primary FRCA. The examiner has been known to give you a plastic skull or an image and ask which foramen is which.

Learning how to draw the base of skull in sections will help you remember the foramina more easily.

## How to draw

### STEP 1

- Draw the bone structure as shown here. The bones are labelled as shown: the frontal bone anteriorly, the temporal bone in the middle and the parietal and occipital bones posteriorly. Between the two frontal bones is the ethmoid bone. The sphenoid bone is central between the frontal bone and the temporal bone, in a butterfly shape. The sella turcica is central to this.

- Draw a big hole in the lower third of the skull. This is the foramen magnum (the biggest hole). This allows the spinal cord, vertebral arteries and the spinal root of the accessory nerve (CN XI) to pass through the skull.

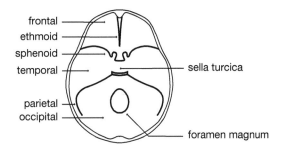

### STEP 2

- Draw a dotted area lateral to the ethmoid bone which represents the cribriform plate (this is part of the ethmoid bone). This is where the olfactory nerve (CN I) passes through the base of skull.

- Draw the optic canal, a small circle anterolateral to the sella turcica. This is where the optic nerve (CN II) passes through the skull.

- The superior orbital fissure is an elliptical shape just along the sphenoid ridge. This is where the oculomotor (CN III), trochlear (CN IV), abducens (CN VI) and the ophthalmic division (V1) of the trigeminal nerve (CN V) pass through the skull.

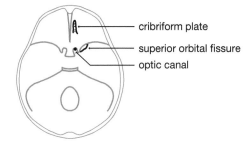

**STEP 3**

- Draw 1 circle, 1 oval-shaped hole and another small circle lateral to the centre of the sphenoid bone, each one slightly lower and further to the right than the last.

- The upper hole is the foramen rotundum (see *Section 1.5: Trigeminal nerve*) where the maxillary branch (V2) of the trigeminal nerve passes.

- The next hole is the foramen ovale, where the mandibular branch (V3) of the trigeminal nerve passes through the skull.

- The third hole is small and is called the foramen spinosum; this is a hole for the middle meningeal artery to pass through.

- The next hole to add is an elliptical shape just lateral to the dorsum sellae. This is the foramen lacerum; it allows the meningeal branches of the ascending pharyngeal artery to pass through the skull.

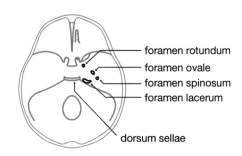

foramen rotundum
foramen ovale
foramen spinosum
foramen lacerum

dorsum sellae

**STEP 4**

- Next you need to draw in 2 small circles and an oval hole laterally (see image for exact positions).

- The hole on the parietal bone ridge is the internal auditory meatus. As suggested in the name, the vestibulocochlear nerve (CN VIII) passes through here, as does the facial nerve (CN VII).

- The larger oval hole is the jugular foramen; 3 cranial nerves pass through here, the glossopharyngeal nerve (CN IX), the vagus nerve (CN X) and the cranial root of the accessory nerve (CN XI).

- The final small hole is the hypoglossal canal and, unsurprisingly, the hypoglossal nerve (CN XII) passes through here.

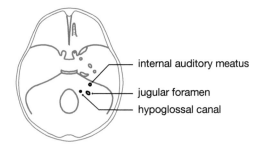

internal auditory meatus

jugular foramen
hypoglossal canal

# 1.5 ▶ Trigeminal nerve

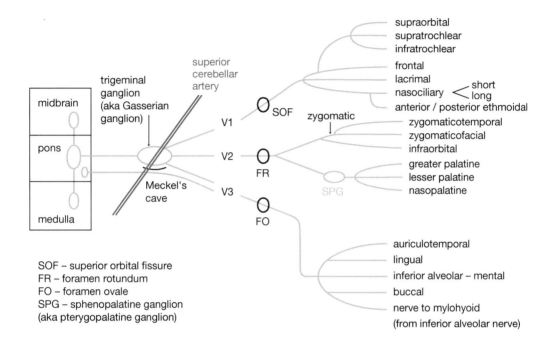

SOF – superior orbital fissure
FR – foramen rotundum
FO – foramen ovale
SPG – sphenopalatine ganglion
(aka pterygopalatine ganglion)

A simple guide to drawing the complicated 5th cranial nerve. By the end of this chapter you will be able to draw up to 18 branches. This will put you miles ahead of anyone else who is asked about the anatomy of the trigeminal nerve.

## How to draw

### STEP 1

Start by drawing the brainstem, where the trigeminal nerve starts.

- Draw a rectangle split into 3 squares. This represents the brainstem – the midbrain, pons and medulla oblongata.

- Draw an arc to represent Meckel's cave.

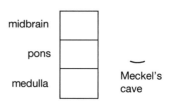

### STEP 2

- Draw 3 sensory nuclei: mesencephalic (midbrain), chief sensory nucleus (pons), and the spinal trigeminal nucleus (medulla). Join the 3 nuclei with straight lines meeting in the middle nucleus.

- Draw the trigeminal ganglion in Meckel's cave.

- Draw one line horizontally to the trigeminal ganglion.

- Draw 3 lines laterally originating at the ganglion; these are the divisions V1, V2 and V3.

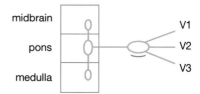

### STEP 3

- Draw an artery across Meckel's cave, to represent that the artery runs near to the trigeminal nerve/ganglion and can cause compression. Compression of the ganglion leading to trigeminal neuralgia is most commonly caused by the superior cerebellar artery (60–90% of the time).

- Draw the motor nucleus in the pons and draw a line that bypasses the ganglion and Meckel's cave. It should run alongside V3.

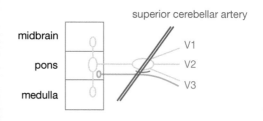

## STEP 4

- From V1 draw one line going through the SOF. This then divides into 3 nerves: the frontal, lacrimal and nasociliary. The frontal nerve gives branches of the supraorbital and supratrochlear. The supratrochlear gives the branch of infratrochlear as shown.

- From the nasociliary nerve draw branches to the anterior and posterior ethmoidal nerves and the branches to the short and long ciliary nerves.

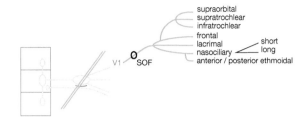

## STEP 5

- Draw a line from V2 that passes through the foramen rotundum and then divides into 2.

- In this simplified version, the upper branch divides into 3 nerves: the infraorbital, the zygomaticotemporal and zygomaticofacial nerves.

- The lower branch forms the sphenopalatine ganglion and then divides into 3; the greater palatine, lesser palatine and nasopalatine nerves.

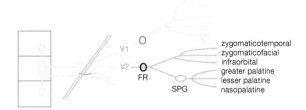

## STEP 6

- Draw a line from V3 that passes through the foramen ovale. It then divides into 5 branches.

- I remember their names by the mnemonic ALIEN (the E is a back to front B in my head!). The branches are the **A**uriculotemporal, **L**ingual, **I**nferior alveolar (mental), **B**uccal and **N**erve to mylohyoid.

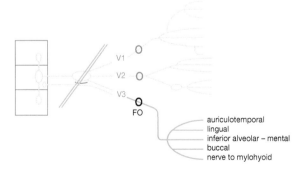

# 1.6 ▶ Motor and sensory innervation of the face

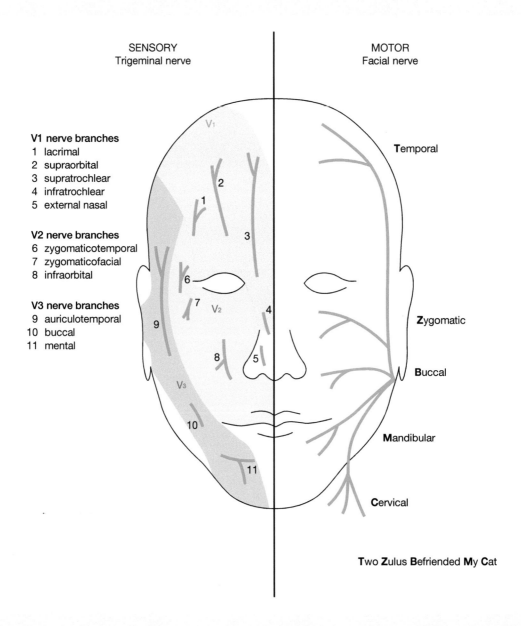

SENSORY
Trigeminal nerve

MOTOR
Facial nerve

**V1 nerve branches**
1 lacrimal
2 supraorbital
3 supratrochlear
4 infratrochlear
5 external nasal

**V2 nerve branches**
6 zygomaticotemporal
7 zygomaticofacial
8 infraorbital

**V3 nerve branches**
9 auriculotemporal
10 buccal
11 mental

V₁

V₂

V₃

**T**emporal

**Z**ygomatic

**B**uccal

**M**andibular

**C**ervical

**T**wo **Z**ulus **B**efriended **M**y **C**at

Sensation to the face arises from the trigeminal nerve (see *Section 1.5: Trigeminal nerve* for branches).

Motor supply to the face is from the facial nerve, cranial nerve VII.

## How to draw

### SENSATION

If you look at the diagram the face can be split into 3 zones: V1, V2 and V3. Each zone has 3–5 branches. Use this image along with the trigeminal nerve diagram to learn the distribution of these nerves.

### MOTOR SUPPLY

The motor supply to facial muscles is from the facial nerve (it's in the name!).

The branches can be remembered using various mnemonics; the one I use is 'Two Zulus Befriended My Cat'. Yes, it is a little odd, but it works for me!

- Temporal nerve: supplies frontalis and procerus muscles.
- Zygomatic: supplies eye and orbit, mid face and smile.
- Buccal: supplies buccinator and upper lips.
- Mandibular: supplies lower lip.
- Cervical: supplies platysma.

# 1.7 ▶ Vagus nerve

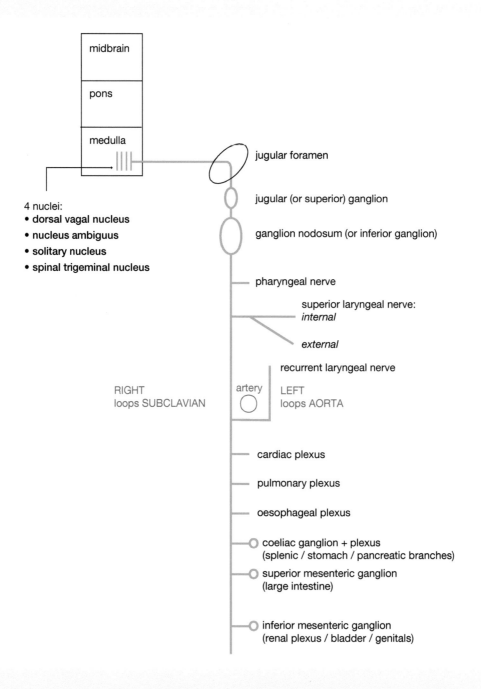

The vagus nerve is a parasympathetic nerve that supplies many organs in
the body. It has been asked about in detail in the SAQ and "viva".

It is a complicated nerve and it runs a different course on each side. The important points are covered in the diagram but I would advise looking on the internet at all the different anatomical images to get a comprehensive and clear idea of where it runs and what it looks like.

There are 4 nuclei in the medulla:

- the dorsal nucleus is the parasympathetic supply to the viscera;

- the nucleus ambiguus is for motor supply;

- the solitary nucleus is for afferent taste;

- the spinal trigeminal nucleus is for deep/crude touch and pain and temperature.

It exits the head through the jugular foramen.

## How to draw

### STEP 1

- Draw the midbrain, pons and medulla as a box.

midbrain

pons

medulla

### STEP 2

- Draw the 4 nuclei (see text above). Draw a line to the right that goes through the jugular foramen and ends in the jugular ganglion. Draw a further line to the ganglion nodosum.

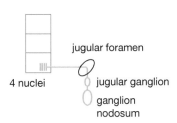

jugular foramen

4 nuclei

jugular ganglion

ganglion nodosum

### STEP 3

Draw a long line down from the ganglion nodosum. Draw 3 branches:

- The superior one is the pharyngeal nerve.

- The next one is the superior laryngeal nerve – this divides into the internal and external branches.

- The third branch represents the recurrent laryngeal nerve – this descends on the left and the right differently. On the right it descends and loops the subclavian artery before ascending into the neck. It lies between the oesophagus and trachea. It supplies sensation below the vocal cords and innervates all of the intrinsic muscles of the larynx except cricothyroid muscle. On the left it descends in the thorax and then loops around the arch of the aorta before ascending.

- Draw the artery, labelled as above.

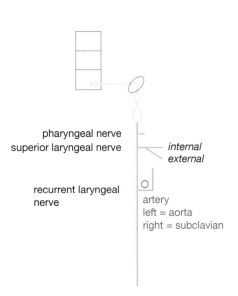

pharyngeal nerve
superior laryngeal nerve

internal
external

recurrent laryngeal nerve

artery
left = aorta
right = subclavian

**STEP 4**

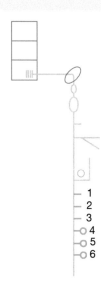

- Draw 4 more branches: these represent the cardiac plexus, pulmonary plexus, oesophageal plexus and the coeliac ganglion and plexus (a circle represents the ganglion).

- Draw 2 further branches – each branch has a circle to represent a ganglion. These are the superior mesenteric ganglion and the inferior mesenteric ganglion.

- The superior mesenteric ganglion has branches to spleen, stomach, pancreas and large intestine.

- The inferior mesenteric ganglion has branches to the renal plexus, bladder and genitals.

1   cardiac plexus
2   pulmonary plexus
3   oesophageal plexus
4   coeliac ganglion + plexus
5   superior mesenteric ganglion
6   inferior mesenteric ganglion

# 1.8 ▸ Cervical plexus

| | |
|---|---|
| **AC** | ansa cervicalis |
| **GA** | greater auricular |
| **LO** | lesser occipital |
| **SC** | supraclavicular |
| **TC** | transverse cervicalis |

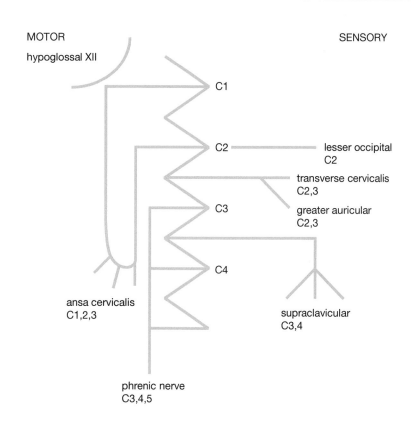

## How to draw

### STEP 1

- Draw 4.5 unfinished arrowheads facing to the right. Label them as C1, 2, 3 and 4.

- C5 is not labelled as it is not 'officially' part of the cervical plexus.

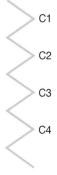

**STEP 2**

Add in the motor component.

- The ansa cervicalis (AC) has roots from C1, 2 and 3 and forms a loop. Three muscles are supplied from the main loop of the ansa cervicalis and this can be represented by drawing 3 lines from the bottom of the loop. (The muscles are: sternohyoid, sternothyroid and omohyoid.)

- Also, draw the phrenic nerve by taking roots from C3, 4 and 5 and joining them together as shown.

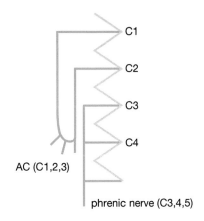

**STEP 3**

Add the sensory nerves to the right side.

- One line from C2 to represent the lesser occipital (LO) nerve.

- One line between C2 and C3 splits into 2. This represents the transverse cervicalis (TC) and greater auricular (GA) nerves.

- Add a third line from between C3 and C4. This will split into 3; the medial, intermediate and lateral supraclavicular (SC) nerves.

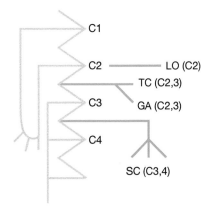

**STEP 4**

- Add in the hypoglossal nerve (CN XII). This carries some motor component of the cervical plexus.

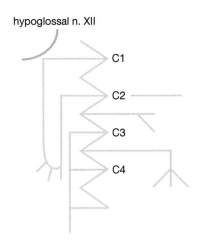

# 1.9 Eye and eye socket bones

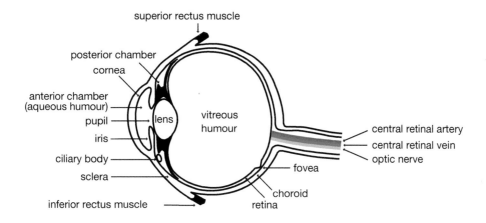

superior rectus muscle

posterior chamber

cornea

anterior chamber
(aqueous humour)

pupil

iris

ciliary body

sclera

inferior rectus muscle

lens

vitreous
humour

central retinal artery

central retinal vein

optic nerve

fovea

choroid

retina

WHAT PASSES THROUGH SUPERIOR ORBITAL FISSURE

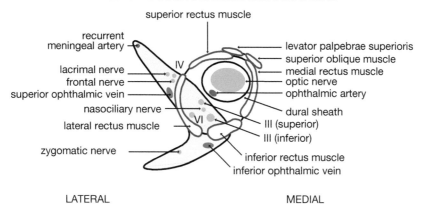

superior rectus muscle

recurrent
meningeal artery

lacrimal nerve

frontal nerve

superior ophthalmic vein

nasociliary nerve

lateral rectus muscle

zygomatic nerve

IV

VI

levator palpebrae superioris

superior oblique muscle

medial rectus muscle

optic nerve

ophthalmic artery

dural sheath

III (superior)

III (inferior)

inferior rectus muscle

inferior ophthalmic vein

LATERAL

MEDIAL

superior orbital fissure

frontal bone (= roof)

optic canal

lesser wing
sphenoid

greater wing
sphenoid

= lateral wall

ethmoidal bone
lacrimal bone

= medial wall

zygoma

maxilla (= floor)

## Nerve supply to the eye

### MOTOR

- III – oculomotor nerve – levator palpebrae muscle, superior rectus muscle, medial rectus muscle and inferior oblique muscle
- IV – trochlear nerve – superior oblique muscle
- VI – abducens nerve – lateral rectus muscle
- VII – facial nerve – orbicularis oculi muscle

### SENSORY

- Trigeminal nerve (CN V)
- V1 (ophthalmic division) – skin / conjunctiva / upper eyelid / between cornea and iris / ciliary muscle / inner eyelid / inner canthus / outer eyelid
- V2 (maxillary division) – lower eyelid / nasolacrimal duct / lateral wall of orbit

### AUTONOMIC

- Sympathetic supply – long and short ciliary nerves from the superior cervical ganglion → these cause iris dilation (mydriasis)
- Parasympathetic supply – fibres from the oculomotor nerve (CN III) → iris constriction (miosis)

## Blood supply

Globe and orbital contents – ophthalmic artery (a branch of the internal carotid artery). The ophthalmic artery passes through the optic canal.

### INTRAOCULAR PRESSURE

Normal intraocular pressure (IOP) is 10–20 mmHg. This increases with age and there is a diurnal variation of 2–3 mmHg.

### AQUEOUS HUMOUR

Clear fluid which fills posterior chamber of the eye. There is approximately 250 μl.

# 2.1 Spinal cord

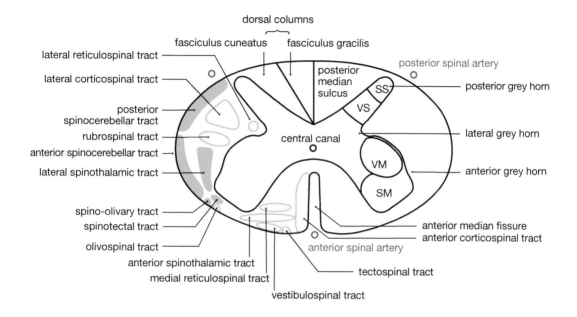

SM somatic motor – consists of interneurons and lower motor neurons that control motor commands to skeletal muscle.

SS somatic sensory – represents the location of the interneurons receiving input from somatic sensory neurons.

VM visceral motor – exists only in the thoracic and upper lumbar region, includes autonomic motor neurons supplying smooth muscle in vessels, viscera and glands. It contains preganglionic visceral motor neurons that project to the sympathetic ganglia.

VS visceral sensory – represents the location of the interneurons receiving input from visceral sensory neurons.

This is a very common question in the primary OSCE; in fact it was one that I was asked. The examiner will often show you an image, they will then point out certain tracts and you need to name them. Both ascending and descending tracts are often on the same side of the image and not always different colours. I have drawn an image with the spinal tracts, ascending and descending, on one side and the cell body/interneurones/motor neurones on the other side. If you learn the method of drawing this then you will be able to label it easily. If the tract starts with 'spino' it is ascending and if it ends with 'spinal' it is descending. Ascending tracts are solid green and descending tracts are green lines only.

**Important points to remember**

The arterial supply to the spinal cord is from 2 posterior spinal arteries and 1 anterior spinal artery. The posterior spinal arteries supply the posterior 1/3 of the spinal cord, and the anterior spinal artery supplies the anterior 2/3 of the spinal cord (see *Section 1.1: Circle of Willis*).

There are 21 paired radicular arteries from the aorta. They all supply the nerve roots and approximately half of them supply the spinal cord by joining the anterior spinal artery. The biggest of them is the artery of Adamkiewicz, which normally originates from L1 region (see *Section 5.1: Abdominal aorta*).

## How to draw

### STEP 1

Draw the main structure:

- the spinal cord shape and a 'butterfly', the grey matter in the middle
- a circle in the middle of the butterfly; this is the central canal
- a line from the top of the butterfly posteriorly – this represents the posterior median sulcus.

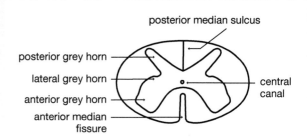

### STEP 2

- Draw the 2 posterior spinal arteries and the anterior spinal artery.

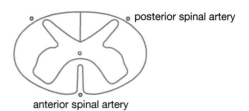

### STEP 3

- Draw 4 lines on one side of the grey matter. Label these parts of the grey matter. In the posterior horn are the somatic sensory (SS) nuclei and visceral sensory (VS) nuclei. In the anterior horn are the visceral motor (VM) nuclei and the somatic motor (SM) nuclei.

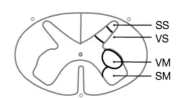

### STEP 4

- Draw a line from the centre at the top of the butterfly diagonally. This represents the dorsal columns, the fasciculus cuneatus laterally and fasciculus gracilis medially.

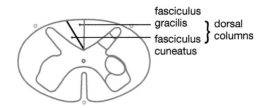

So for the main section…. Start by drawing along the edge, posteriorly to anteriorly. First draw:

- 2 large tracts – these are the posterior spinocerebellar and anterior spinocerebellar tracts

- 2 small tracts – these are the olivospinal and spino-olivary tracts.

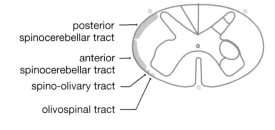

posterior spinocerebellar tract

anterior spinocerebellar tract

spino-olivary tract

olivospinal tract

Then draw 3 more tracts finishing just along the anterior median fissure:

- 1 large tract to the right of the olivospinal and spino-olivary tracts – this is the anterior spinothalamic tract

- 1 small tract – the tectospinal tract

- 1 further large tract – the anterior corticospinal tract.

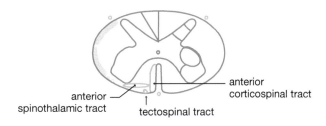

anterior spinothalamic tract

tectospinal tract

anterior corticospinal tract

- Add in 2 slightly larger tracts just posteriorly to the tectospinal tract; these are the vestibulospinal and medial reticulospinal tracts.

- Then add in one small tract just behind the olivospinal and spino-olivary tracts; this is the spinotectal tract.

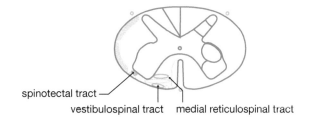

spinotectal tract

vestibulospinal tract     medial reticulospinal tract

Draw 4 tracts medially to the outer edge, going backwards as shown.

- The most posterior one is the lateral corticospinal tract; this is the biggest.

lateral corticospinal tract

rubrospinal tract

lateral reticulospinal tract

lateral spinothalamic tract

- The middle one is the rubrospinal tract.

- The one in front of this is the lateral spinothalamic tract.

- In the narrowing of the wing of the butterfly is the lateral reticulospinal tract.

An important point to note is that when pain proceduralists do spinothalamic tract radio frequency ablation it is in very close proximity to the rubrospinal tract and so if this is accidentally damaged, the patient would suffer weakness in the diaphragm.

# 2.2 Epidural space

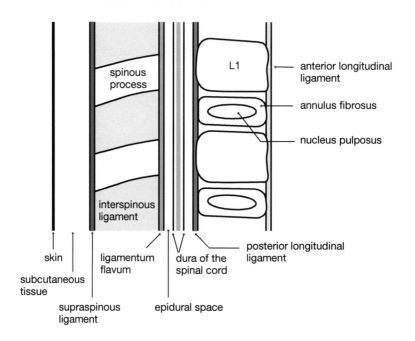

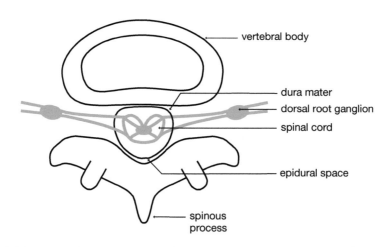

This diagram is important to learn because you will commonly be asked about the anatomy of the epidural space at work and in the exam. The illustrations simplify the anatomy so you can imagine what it would look like in a sagittal and a horizontal cross-section.

**What layers would your needle pass through to get to the epidural space?**
Answer: from the outside to inside: skin, subcutaneous tissue, supraspinous ligament, interspinous ligament and ligamentum flavum.

**What is contained in the epidural space?**
Answer: epidural fat, lymphatics, dural sac, spinal nerves, spinal arteries and epidural venous plexus.

## How to draw

### STEP 1

- Draw 1 single and 1 pair of longitudinal lines approximately 2 cm apart.

- Draw L1 and L2 vertebrae – in between the vertebrae draw the vertebral discs.

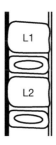

### STEP 2

- Draw 3 vertical lines; the middle one is the spinal cord (green).

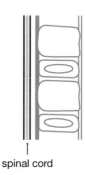

spinal cord

**STEP 3**

- Draw the ligamentum flavum and then the 2 spinous processes.

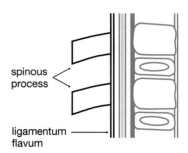

spinous process

ligamentum flavum

**STEP 4**

- Draw 4 more vertical lines. The layers are (deep to superficial): interspinous ligament, supraspinous ligament, subcutaneous tissue and skin.

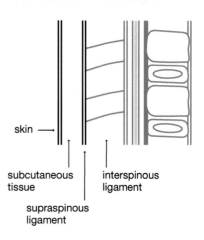

skin

subcutaneous tissue

interspinous ligament

supraspinous ligament

# 2.3 Paravertebral space

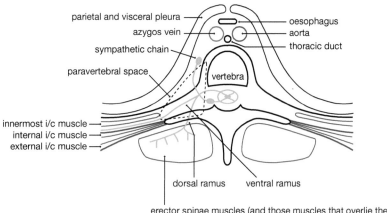

parietal and visceral pleura — oesophagus
azygos vein — aorta
sympathetic chain — thoracic duct
paravertebral space — vertebra
innermost i/c muscle —
internal i/c muscle —
external i/c muscle —
dorsal ramus      ventral ramus
erector spinae muscles (and those muscles that overlie them)

This is a complicated area. If you break it down it becomes easier to draw. If you can draw it then you should be able to label it for the exam (though they shouldn't expect you to draw it!).

## How to draw

### STEP 1

• Draw the vertebral body as shown.

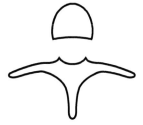

**STEP 2**

- Draw 2 oval/square shapes behind the vertebra and lateral to it (as shown). These represent the erector spinae and the latissimus dorsi muscles.

- Draw 4 lines coming out of the transverse process of the vertebrae. These are the external and internal intercostal muscles (at the posterior aspect, the internal intercostal muscles are replaced by the internal intercostal membranes). Draw the innermost intercostal muscle just anterior to these.

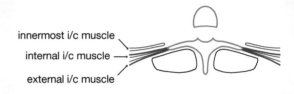

**STEP 3**

- Draw a line that is anterior to the innermost intercostal muscle and the vertebral body; this is the endothoracic fascia.

- Just in front of this draw the parietal and visceral pleura.

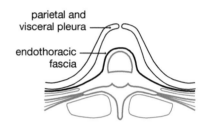

**STEP 4**

- Draw 1 red circle (aorta), one blue circle (azygos vein), 1 black circle (thoracic duct) and 1 black lozenge (oesophagus) just anterior to the vertebral body.

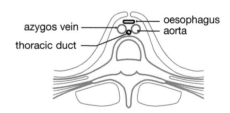

**STEP 5**

- Draw the simplified version of the spinal cord and branches as shown.

- The dorsal and ventral roots join to form the spinal nerve. The spinal nerve communicates with the sympathetic trunk by the white and grey rami communicantes. The spinal nerve divides into the ventral and dorsal rami. The ventral ramus in the thoracic region is known as the intercostal nerve. The dorsal rami travel to innervate the skin and muscles of the back.

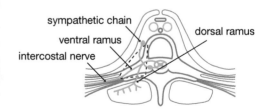

# 2.4 Vertebrae

**Cervical** — most have a bifid spine

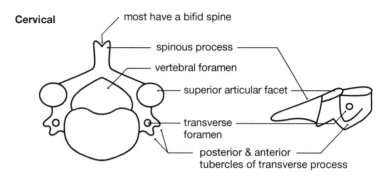

- spinous process
- vertebral foramen
- superior articular facet
- transverse foramen
- posterior & anterior tubercles of transverse process

**Thoracic**

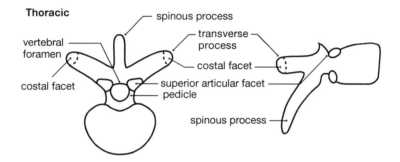

- spinous process
- transverse process
- vertebral foramen
- costal facet
- costal facet
- superior articular facet
- pedicle
- spinous process

**Lumbar**

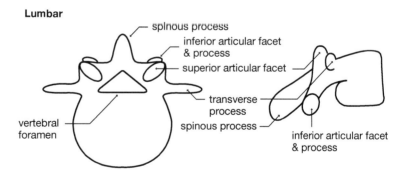

- spinous process
- inferior articular facet & process
- superior articular facet
- transverse process
- vertebral foramen
- spinous process
- inferior articular facet & process

**View from above**          **View from the side**

## The difference between cervical, thoracic and lumbar vertebrae

Here are a few notes to help. It is also a good idea to research on the internet the differences between the vertebrae. There are some lovely tables that will help you to differentiate.

### CERVICAL VERTEBRAE

These are the smallest vertebrae. Each has 3 foramina – 1 vertebral and 2 transverse. The cervical vertebra is fairly flat when you look at it from the side. The first and second cervical vertebrae are quite different (as you should know!).

### THORACIC VERTEBRAE

Thoracic vertebrae are bigger than cervical vertebrae but smaller than lumbar vertebrae. They only have 1 vertebral foramen. The spinous processes are longer and thicker than cervical vertebrae and they are at a larger angle, directed caudally. The transverse processes are quite large. When you look down on the main body and processes it looks a bit like a T-shape.

### LUMBAR VERTEBRAE

These are the biggest vertebrae. They also have only 1 vertebral foramen. When you look down on them they look like they have 5 projections due to the facet joints.

# 2.5 Sacrum and sacral anatomy

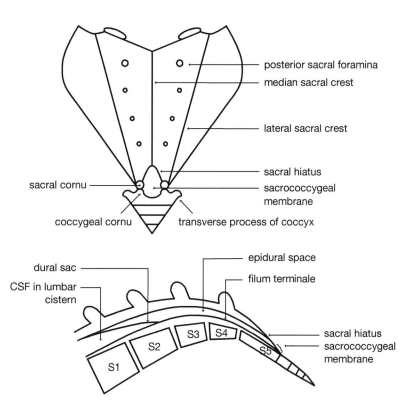

It is important to understand in your mind what the sagittal cross-section of the sacral canal looks like. This is for practical purposes and examination purposes!

The bony anatomy of the sacrum can also be asked and is fairly simple so try to learn these two diagrams so you will not be caught out. You may be asked to perform a caudal on a model (I was!).

## Common questions

**What is contained in the caudal space?**
Answer: the volume is normally 30–35 ml in an adult. It contains epidural fat, sacral nerves, lymphatics, the filum terminale and the venous plexus.

**What dosing of local anaesthetic is required in the paediatric population?**
Answer: in paediatrics local anaesthetic dose is based on the weight of the child and the height of the block you want.

The Armitage formula is used to determine dosing of levobupivacaine 0.25% (in ml/kg):

| | |
|---|---|
| Sacrolumbar block | 0.5 ml/kg |
| Upper abdominal block | 1 ml/kg |
| Mid thoracic block | 1.25 ml/kg |

# 3.1 Coronary arteries

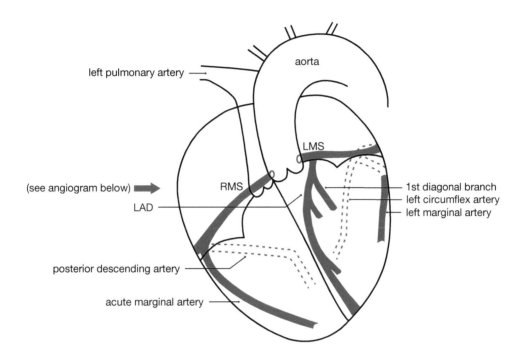

left pulmonary artery

aorta

LMS

(see angiogram below)

RMS

1st diagonal branch
left circumflex artery
left marginal artery

LAD

posterior descending artery

acute marginal artery

LAD    left anterior descending artery
LMS    left main stem
RMS    right main stem

- The two coronary ostia arise from the sinuses of Valsalva just above the aortic valve.

- The left coronary artery starts as the left main stem. It then divides into the left anterior descending (LAD) artery and circumflex artery. The LAD has diagonal arteries coming off it and supplies the interventricular septum and the lateral and anterior walls of the left ventricle.

- The circumflex artery winds around the back of the heart. The posterior descending artery is from the right coronary artery in 85% of people (right dominant) and from the circumflex artery in 15% of people (left dominant). The circumflex artery supplies the posterior and lateral side of the left ventricle. The left marginal (or obtuse) artery branches from the circumflex.

- The right coronary artery starts as the right main stem and divides into the acute marginal artery (anteriorly) and the posterior descending artery (posteriorly). These supply the right ventricle.

Sometimes you are shown an angiogram. This can be a bit of a trick question; most people think an angiogram has the circumflex running along the top of the image. However, the most common view looks at a sagittal cross-section through the heart and hence the LAD is along the top of the image.

**Angiogram**
Looks from RIGHT lateral,
see red arrow in main drawing

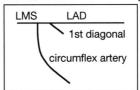

# 3.2 Venous drainage of the heart

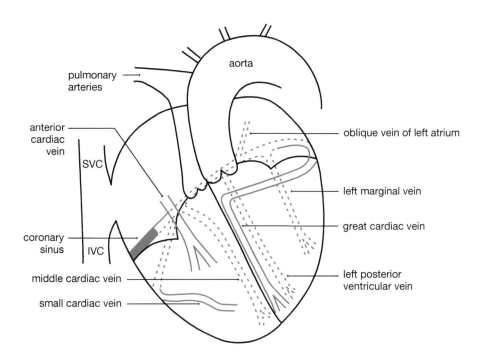

pulmonary arteries

aorta

anterior cardiac vein

oblique vein of left atrium

SVC

left marginal vein

great cardiac vein

coronary sinus

IVC

middle cardiac vein

left posterior ventricular vein

small cardiac vein

IVC    inferior vena cava
SVC    superior vena cava

- Cardiac veins often follow the course of the coronary arteries. They mainly drain into the coronary sinus located in the right atrium between the IVC and the tricuspid valve.

- There are 2–5 anterior cardiac veins that receive blood from the right ventricle and pass the coronary sinus to empty directly into the right atrium (one drawn in the image above as an example).

- Thebesian veins are small and directly drain into the chambers of the heart. They account for true shunt.

# 4.1 Airway sensation

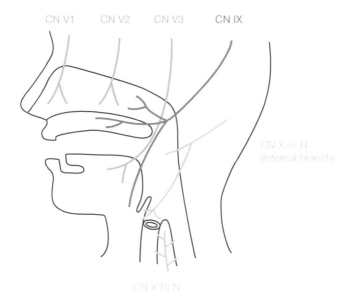

CN V1    CN V2    CN V3    CN IX

CN X SLN
(internal branch)

CN X RLN

CN V    trigeminal nerve
    CN V1 – anterior ethmoidal nerve
    CN V2 – sphenopalatine nerve
    CN V3 – lingual nerve
CN IX    glossopharyngeal nerve
CN X    vagus nerve
    CN X RLN – recurrent laryngeal nerve
    CN X SLN – superior laryngeal nerve

To answer the question:

*"Which nerves do you need to anaesthetise for an awake fibreoptic intubation (AFOI)?"*

you need to know the diagram above.

Airway sensation is from cranial nerves V, IX and X.

## TRIGEMINAL NERVE, CN V

- V1 branch: the anterior ethmoidal nerve; innervates the septum and nasal cavity.

- V2 branch: the sphenopalatine, greater and lesser palatine nerves. The greater palatine nerve innervates the gums and the mucous membrane of the hard palate. The lesser palatine nerve innervates the nasal cavity, the soft palate, the tonsils and the uvula.

- V3 branch: the lingual nerve; sensory innervation of the tongue.

### GLOSSOPHARYNGEAL NERVE, CN IX

- Sensory innervation to upper pharynx and posterior third of the tongue.

### VAGUS NERVE, CN X

- Superior laryngeal nerve: sensory innervation to the lower pharynx, epiglottis, vallecula and piriform fossa.
- Recurrent laryngeal nerve: sensation to the vocal cord and subglottic mucosa.

# 4.2 Larynx

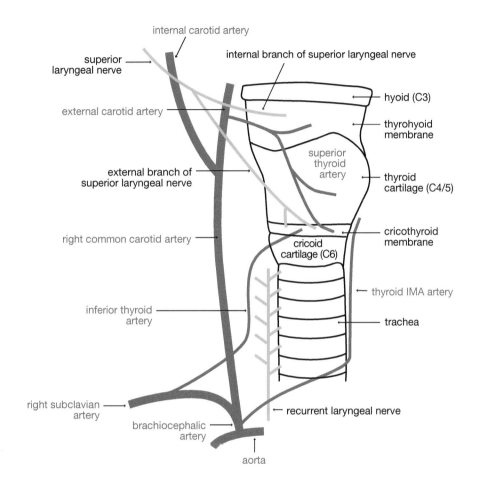

internal carotid artery

superior laryngeal nerve

internal branch of superior laryngeal nerve

external carotid artery

external branch of superior laryngeal nerve

right common carotid artery

inferior thyroid artery

right subclavian artery

brachiocephalic artery

aorta

hyoid (C3)

thyrohyoid membrane

superior thyroid artery

thyroid cartilage (C4/5)

cricothyroid membrane

cricoid cartilage (C6)

thyroid IMA artery

trachea

recurrent laryngeal nerve

## How to draw

STEP 1

Draw the main structures in black pen.

- Start with the trachea, a rectangle shape with lines to represent the cartilage rings (c-shaped).

- Then add in the cricoid cartilage by drawing a trapezium above the trachea (see image). The cricoid cartilage is actually slightly larger at the back than the front, in the shape of a signet ring.

- Next draw an irregular polygon to represent the thyrohyoid membrane, thyroid cartilage and cricothyroid membrane.

- Draw 2 lines inside this to separate the 3 structures.

- Draw the hyoid bone as a rounded rectangle above the thyrohyoid membrane.

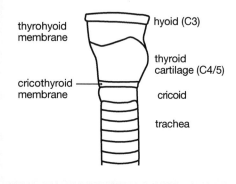

STEP 2

- Draw the superior laryngeal nerve (SLN), a branch of the vagus nerve (CN X). The SLN branches from the vagus nerve at approximately C2. It then divides into the internal branch and external branch at the level of hyoid (C3).

- The internal branch pierces the thyrohyoid membrane with the superior laryngeal artery. It supplies sensation to the mucosa above the vocal cords.

- The external branch supplies the cricothyroid muscle (see where it ends on the diagram).

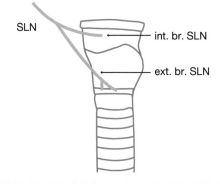

STEP 3

- Draw in the recurrent laryngeal nerve, a branch of the vagus nerve. It runs in the groove between the oesophagus and the trachea and supplies sensation to the mucosa of the larynx below the vocal cords. It also innervates most of the intrinsic muscles of the pharynx except the cricothyroid muscle.

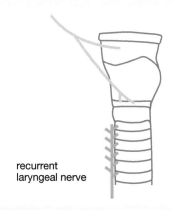

- Draw in the arch of the aorta inferiorly. The brachiocephalic artery arises here and then divides into the right subclavian artery and the right common carotid artery.

- The common carotid artery ascends and divides into the internal and external carotid arteries at the level of the thyroid cartilage (approximately C4).

- The left carotid and left subclavian arteries arise directly from the aortic arch (not shown here).

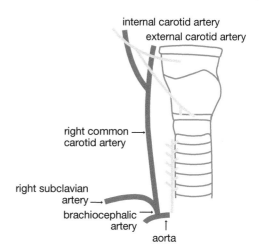

internal carotid artery
external carotid artery
right common carotid artery
right subclavian artery
brachiocephalic artery
aorta

- Draw in the inferior thyroid artery, a branch of the thyrocervical trunk which arises from the right subclavian artery.

- Draw in the superior thyroid artery, a branch of the external carotid artery (at approximately C3). Finally draw in the thyroid IMA artery, a variable branch of the brachiocephalic artery. This artery is only present in 3–10% of the population. It can be the reason for bleeding during a tracheostomy.

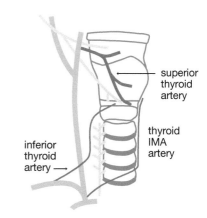

superior thyroid artery
thyroid IMA artery
inferior thyroid artery

# 4.3 Laryngoscopic view of the vocal cords

G   glottis

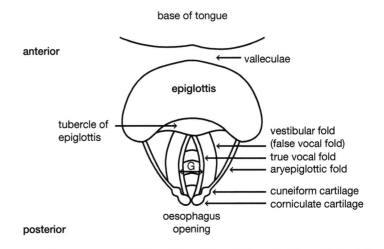

base of tongue

anterior

← valleculae

epiglottis

tubercle of epiglottis

vestibular fold (false vocal fold)

true vocal fold

aryepiglottic fold

cuneiform cartilage

corniculate cartilage

oesophagus opening

posterior

Looking through the mouth at the larynx with a laryngoscope is an essential skill for an anaesthetist. Being able to describe exactly what you can see will show the consultant anaesthetist that you know what you are looking at, and it may give you a bit more time to intubate before they take over.

The image above shows exactly what you will see, the tongue base superiorly and the corniculate cartilage (in front of the oesophagus) posteriorly.

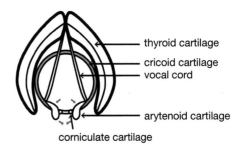

thyroid cartilage

cricoid cartilage

vocal cord

arytenoid cartilage

corniculate cartilage

This image shows what the view would look like with no soft tissue and shows how the cartilage is moved to open and close the vocal cords.

N.B. Anaesthetists often refer to the corniculate cartilage as 'the arytenoids'. As you can see this is technically the corniculate and cuneiform cartilage.

## Nerve supply to the larynx

The nervous supply to the larynx is by the external branch of the superior laryngeal nerve above the cords and the recurrent laryngeal nerve below. Both are branches of the vagus nerve (CN X).

The external branch of the superior laryngeal nerve only supplies cricothyroid muscle and the recurrent laryngeal nerve supplies all other muscles of the larynx. Hence, damage to the recurrent laryngeal nerve can lead to vocal cord palsy.

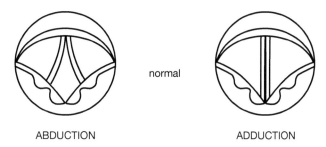

normal

ABDUCTION                    ADDUCTION

The vocal cords are used to generate sound by vibration of air passing between the adducted cords. Abducted cords are for breathing/breathy sounds and whispering. The vocal cords oscillate due to increased pressure beneath the vocal folds. The lower part of the vocal cords move before the upper part and this creates a wave-like motion. The pitch of a person's voice depends on length, size and tension of their vocal cords.

## Superior laryngeal nerve damage

- The external branch may be damaged during thyroid surgery.
- It supplies cricothyroid muscle.
- Damage leads to a loss of vocal cord tensions and hence a hoarse voice.
- If unilateral the other side often compensates.

## Recurrent laryngeal nerve damage

This is also known as vocal cord paresis and this can cause bilateral and unilateral paralysis as shown over the page.

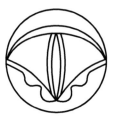
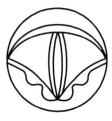

bilateral
paralysis

RESPIRATION                    PHONATION

- Complete transection of the nerve causes complete paralysis of most muscles except cricothyroid (innervated by the superior laryngeal nerve).
- This leads to a half abducted, half adducted position – the cadaveric position.
- **Symptoms:** patient cannot speak or cough.

- Trauma/partial transection leads to partial paralysis.
- This leaves the cords in an adducted position.
- **Symptoms:** respiratory distress, stridor, life threatening.

UNILATERAL DAMAGE

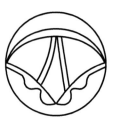
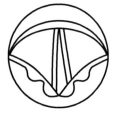

unilateral
paralysis

RESPIRATION                    PHONATION

- If one cord is damaged then the other cord will partially compensate.
- The damaged cord will sit in an adducted position as cricothyroid muscle should still work (due to innervation by the superior laryngeal nerve).
- **Symptoms:** breathy voice, weak cough, sensation of shortness of breath and sometimes swallowing difficulties.

# 4.4 Bronchial tree

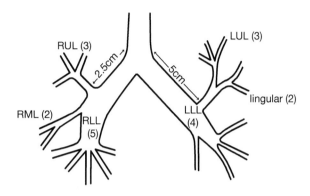

| | | | | |
|---|---|---|---|---|
| LLL | - left lower lobe | **19 Segments** | - Right | - upper - 3 |
| LUL | - left upper lobe | | | - middle - 2 |
| RLL | - right lower lobe | | | - lower - 5 |
| RML | - right middle lobe | | | **10** |
| RUL | - right upper lobe | | | |
| | | | - Left | - upper - 3 |
| | | | | - lingular - 2 |
| | | | | - lower - 4 |
| | | | | **9** |

This is a common topic for a question. Learning to draw the diagram is not important, but knowing the number of segments and their names is useful.

I remember it as '325, 324'. This adds up to 19 segments in total, 10 on the right and 9 on the left.

The right main bronchus is approximately 2.5 cm long and straight, about 25° off the midline.

The left main bronchus is approximately 5 cm long and lies more horizontally over the heart, about 45° off the midline.

RIGHT SIDE

- 3: APA – Apical, Posterior, Anterior
- 2: LM: Lateral, Medial
- 5: APALM: Apical, Posterior, Anterior, Lateral, Medial

LEFT SIDE

- 3: APA – Apical, Posterior, Anterior
- 2: IS – Inferior, Superior (LINGULAR)
- 4: APAL – Apical, Posterior, Anterior, Lateral (there is no medial one – this can be remembered by thinking that the heart lies where it would have been!)

# 4.5 Thoracic inlet

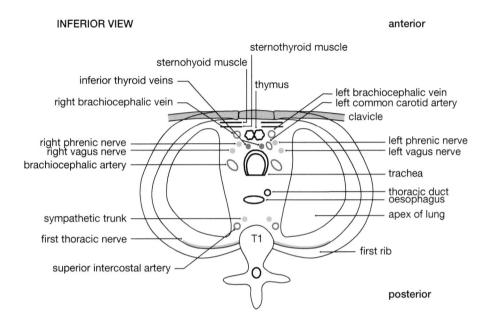

INFERIOR VIEW                                                anterior

- sternothyroid muscle
- sternohyoid muscle
- inferior thyroid veins
- right brachiocephalic vein
- thymus
- left brachiocephalic vein
- left common carotid artery
- clavicle
- right phrenic nerve
- right vagus nerve
- brachiocephalic artery
- left phrenic nerve
- left vagus nerve
- trachea
- thoracic duct
- oesophagus
- apex of lung
- sympathetic trunk
- first thoracic nerve
- T1
- first rib
- superior intercostal artery

posterior

Another exam favourite!

This is a complicated area; it basically means "what is at the level of the 1st rib?".

## How to draw

**STEP 1**

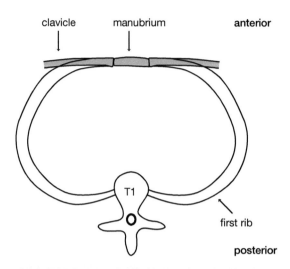

INFERIOR VIEW

clavicle     manubrium     anterior

T1

first rib

posterior

- Draw an oval shape with T1 in the centre at the back.
- Draw a second oval inside this; the outer area is the first rib.
- Draw a straight line at the front that represents the manubrium and the clavicle.

**STEP 2**

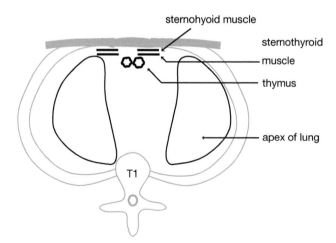

sternohyoid muscle

sternothyroid muscle

thymus

apex of lung

T1

- Draw an enclosed semicircle on each side to represent the apex of each lung. Draw 2 sets of small parallel lines at the front just behind the manubrium. These are the sternohyoid and sternothyroid muscles. Just behind these draw two little fluffy cloud shapes to represent the thymus.

STEP 3

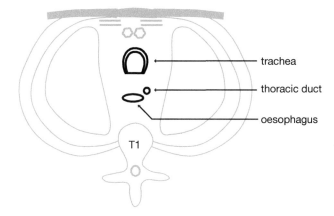

- Add in a trachea behind the thymus and then draw the oesophagus and thoracic duct behind the trachea.

STEP 4

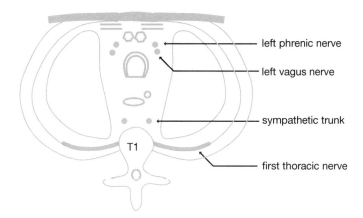

- Draw 2 green lines from T1 to just in front of the posterior first rib; these represent the first thoracic nerves.
- Draw 2 green dots anterior to T1 body; these are the sympathetic trunks.
- Draw 2 green dots just in front of and lateral to the trachea; these are the right and left vagus nerves.
- Draw 2 green dots just in front of the vagus nerves; these are the phrenic nerves.

**STEP 5**

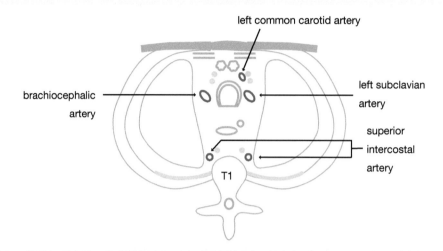

left common carotid artery

brachiocephalic artery

left subclavian artery

superior intercostal artery

T1

- Draw 2 red circles just lateral and behind the sympathetic trunks; these are the superior intercostal arteries.

- Draw 2 red ovals lateral to the trachea; these represent the brachiocephalic artery and the left subclavian artery.

- Draw a red circle just anterior to the left subclavian artery and medial to the phrenic and vagus nerves; this is the left common carotid artery.

**STEP 6**

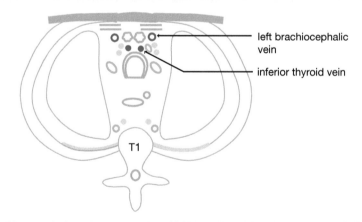

left brachiocephalic vein

inferior thyroid vein

T1

- Draw 2 blue dots just in front of the trachea; these are the inferior thyroid veins.

- Draw 2 blue circles anterior to these and lateral to the thymus; these are the brachiocephalic veins.

## 4.6 First rib

posterior

articular facet with T1 vertebrae
(most ribs have 2 but the first only has 1)

tubercle

HEAD

external/internal intercostal
muscle insertion

sympathetic trunk

T1 nerve

supreme i/c vein

scalenus medius muscle insertion

superior i/c artery

serratus anterior muscle insertion

scalene tubercle
(scalenus anterior muscle insertion)

subclavian artery

suprapleural membrane

subclavian groove
subclavian vein

subclavius

costoclavicular ligament

anterior

Sometimes in the exam you are handed the first rib (plastic version) and asked to explain which way up it lies and what runs in what groove.

The under surface of the first rib is smoother. If you lay the rib on the table you can see it is the correct way up as the head will touch the surface.

The image shows the superior surface of the first rib. It is important to know where the vessels run over the rib.

If you find the scalenus tubercle (for scalenus anterior) then you will find the subclavian groove.

- The subclavian artery runs posteriorly to this and the subclavian vein runs anteriorly.

- The T1 nerve root runs under the subclavian artery.

# 4.7 ▶ Intercostal nerves

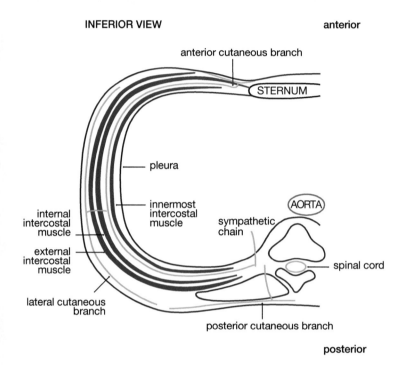

The intercostal nerves arise from the anterior rami of the thoracic nerves T1 to T11. The upper 2 nerves supply the upper limb and the thorax. The next 4 nerves supply the thorax and the lower 5 nerves supply the thorax and abdominal walls. The 7th intercostal nerve terminates at the xiphoid process and the 10th intercostal nerve terminates at the navel.

## How to draw

**STEP 1**

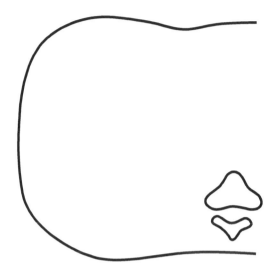

- Draw an approximate semicircle to represent the thorax and then draw one of the thoracic vertebrae (in two halves, the body and the spinous processes).

**STEP 2**

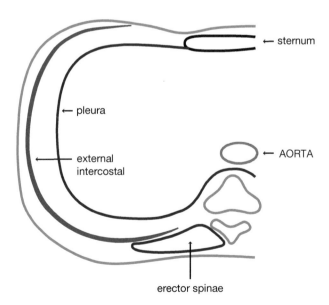

- Add in the external intercostal muscle by drawing a brown semicircle from the transverse process anteriorly. Draw the erector spinae muscle.
- Draw the pleura, anterior to the thoracic vertebral body and ending by drawing the sternum. Add the aorta anterior to the pleura.

**STEP 3**

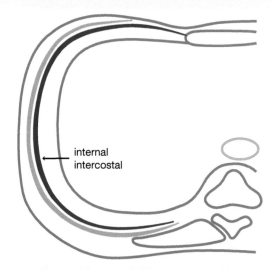

- Draw the internal intercostal muscle by drawing a semicircular line from the transverse process to the sternum.

**STEP 4**

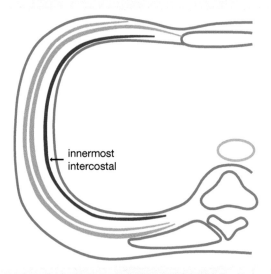

- Draw the innermost intercostal muscle by drawing a semicircular line just inside the pleura.

STEP 5

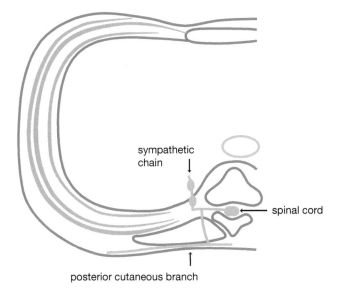

sympathetic chain

spinal cord

posterior cutaneous branch

- Draw the spinal cord in between the body of the vertebrae and the spinous process.
- Draw the sympathetic chain anteriorly and the posterior cutaneous nerve posteriorly.

STEP 6

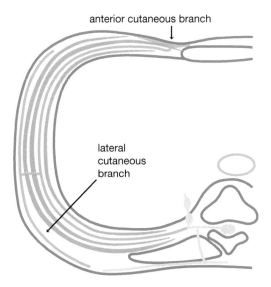

anterior cutaneous branch

lateral cutaneous branch

- As a new branch from the spinal nerve, draw a semicircular nerve between the innermost and internal intercostal muscles. Finish it anteriorly with an anterior cutaneous branch.
- Draw a lateral cutaneous branch from the anterior branch as shown.

# 4.8 Mediastinum

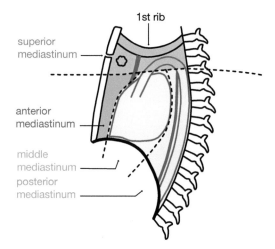

The mediastinum has been known to come up in the FRCA and so it is an important area to know.

The mediastinum is divided into the:

- superior mediastinum
- anterior mediastinum
- middle mediastinum
- posterior mediastinum

You should also know a cross-section anatomy through approximately T6 (anterior, middle and posterior) as this has also been asked about.

### ANTERIOR MEDIASTINUM

- This contains loose connective tissue, fat, lymphatic vessels, lymph nodes and branches of internal thoracic vessels.
- The thymus sometimes extends inferiorly into the anterior mediastinum.

### MIDDLE MEDIASTINUM

- This contains major organs and vessels including the heart, ascending aorta, pulmonary trunk, superior vena cava, pericardium, tracheal bifurcation and left and right main bronchi.
- There are also tracheobronchial lymph nodes.

## POSTERIOR MEDIASTINUM

- This is where the thoracic descending aorta lies. Branches that come off the aorta here are the posterior intercostal arteries, bronchial arteries, oesophageal arteries and superior phrenic arteries.

- The oesophagus, thoracic duct, azygos vein, hemiazygos vein and sympathetic trunks lie here.

## SUPERIOR MEDIASTINUM

- Major blood vessels are in this part of the mediastinum, including the arch of aorta and branches (brachiocephalic, left common carotid, left subclavian artery), the superior vena cava, left and right brachiocephalic veins, supreme intercostal vein and azygos vein.

- Nerves here are the right and left vagus nerves, phrenic nerves, cardiac nerves and sympathetic trunk.

- Other structures include the thymus, trachea, thoracic duct, sternohyoid and sternothyroid muscles.

# 4.9 Diaphragm

A    right phrenic
     nerve
B    vagal trunks
C    left gastric
     vessels
D    aorta
E    thoracic duct
F    hemiazygos vein

IVC  inferior vena
     cava

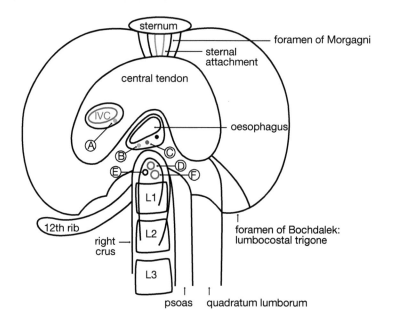

This would not be easy to draw in an exam but it does get asked about. This is the simplest version of the diaphragm that I could come up with.

The main things to learn are what passes through where and the nerve supply.

The motor supply of the diaphragm is from the left and right phrenic nerves (C3, 4 and 5). The phrenic nerve also supplies sensation to the central tendon. The sensation at the edge of the diaphragm is from the intercostal nerves T5 to T12.

The right crus of the diaphragm arises from L1 to L3. The left crus arises from L1 to L2.

Caval opening: **T8**

- Vena cava (**8** letters)
- R phrenic (**8** letters) nerve

Oesophageal opening: **T10**

- Oesophagus (**10** letters)
- Vagal trunk (cranial nerve **10**)
- Left gastric vessels

Aortic hiatus (**12** letters): **T12**

- Aorta
- Thoracic duct (**12** letters)
- Azygos vein

# 5.1 Abdominal aorta

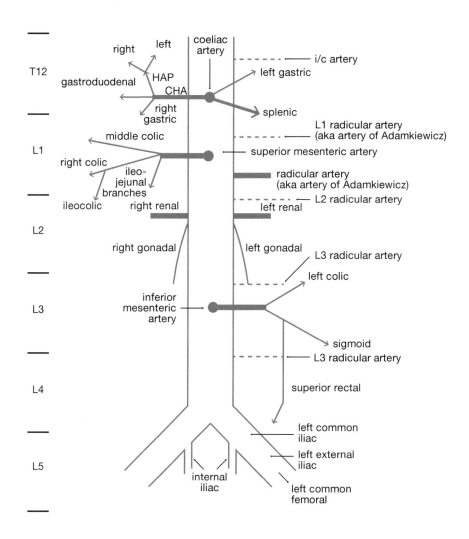

| | |
|---|---|
| CHA | common hepatic artery |
| HAP | hepatic artery proper |
| i/c | intercostal |
| IMA | inferior mesenteric artery |
| SMA | superior mesenteric artery |

This has come up in the exam before.

## How to draw

- Label the levels from T12 to L5, evenly spaced down the page.

- Draw the aorta. The bifurcation into the two common iliac veins is at the L4 level.

- From the common iliac vessels draw a line downwards on each side; these represent the internal iliac arteries.

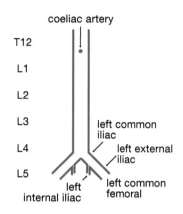

- The coeliac artery branches from the aorta at the T12/L1 level. Draw a horizontal line through the aorta that bifurcates at the left end and splits into 4 on the right side.

- The left side becomes the left gastric and splenic arteries.

- The right side becomes the hepatic (left and right) arteries, the gastroduodenal artery and the right gastric artery.

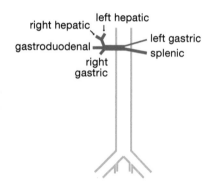

- Just inferior to the coeliac plexus (and to the right side, just for ease) draw the superior mesenteric artery. This divides into the middle colic, right colic, ileocolic and ileojejunal arteries.

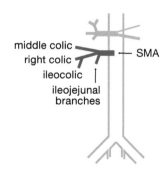

STEP 4

- Between L1/2 level, draw a horizontal line which represents the left and right renal arteries.

- Diagonally downwards from L2 level are the gonadal arteries.

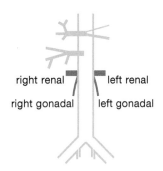

STEP 5

- At approximately L3, draw the inferior mesenteric artery (IMA; to the left). This branches into the left colic artery and the sigmoid artery. The superior rectal artery is a continuation of the IMA.

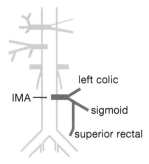

STEP 6

- Finally, draw some dotted lines at each level to represent the intercostal artery and lumbar radicular arteries.

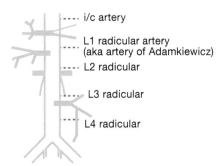

# 5.2 Coeliac plexus

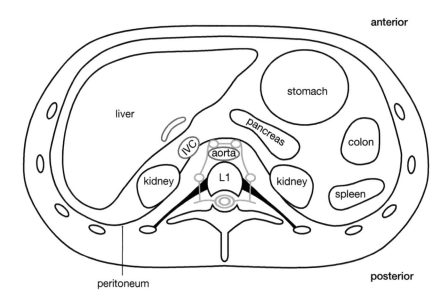

anterior

posterior

peritoneum

| | | | | |
|---|---|---|---|---|
| C | colon | L | liver |
| IVC | inferior vena cava | P | pancreas |
| K | kidney | Sp | spleen |

This diagram is drawn with the lumbar vertebrae at the top of the drawing and can be imagined looking at the patient from the feet towards the head.

The coeliac plexus is also known as the solar plexus. It is the main autonomic nerve supply to intraabdominal organs. Performing a coeliac plexus nerve block, at L1, can help alleviate chronic pain caused by specific organs, e.g. pancreatitis-related pain.

Sympathetic supply is from the splanchnic nerves and parasympathetic supply is from the vagus nerves (cranial nerve 10).

The peritoneum is made up of the parietal peritoneum (lines the body wall) and the visceral peritoneum (lines the abdominal viscera). This is not depicted in the diagram to avoid making it too complicated. Organs are often described as intraperitoneal or retroperitoneal. Retroperitoneal organs have peritoneum on their anterior side only. Retroperitoneal organs include adrenal glands, duodenum (2nd and 3rd segments), pancreas, both kidneys and ureters, ascending and descending colon, oesophagus, rectum, aorta and inferior vena cava. Intraperitoneal organs include the stomach, spleen, liver, bulb of the duodenum, jejunum, ileum, sigmoid colon and transverse colon. Some people use mnemonics to remember which organs are retroperitoneal – check online for memory aids!

## How to draw

### STEP 1

- Draw an oval shape to represent the cross-section of the body.

- Draw one vertebra in the middle, ideally drawn with the main body and spinous processes separately (label it L1).

- Add 5 small ovals around each side to represent the end of the ribs that may be seen in cross-section.

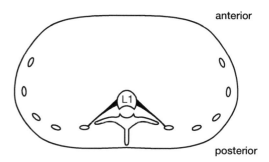

### STEP 2

- Draw the peritoneum as one large kidney bean shape (on its side).

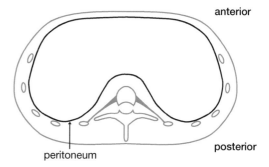

### STEP 3

- Add in the organs; 2 kidneys (one either side of the L1 main body), the pancreas (just in front of L1), the stomach (anterior to the pancreas), the spleen and colon (lateral to the stomach) and the liver (the biggest organ in front of the right kidney).

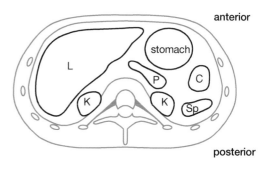

### STEP 4

- The aorta lies anteriorly to the L1 main body and posteriorly to the peritoneum. Draw a blue oval to represent the IVC which lies just anteriorly to the peritoneum.

- Draw the coeliac plexus as a green structure which encircles the L1 body and aorta. The 2 circles lateral to L1 main body are the sympathetic chain; the 2 anterior to the aorta are the coeliac plexus; the 1 behind the vertebral body is the spinal cord.

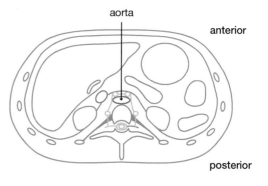

# 5.3 Abdominal wall

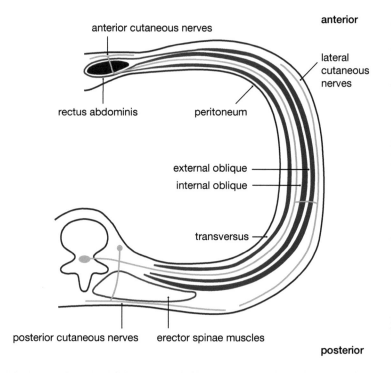

This is a similar diagram to the intercostal nerves. However, the difference is that the three muscles from inner to outer are the:

- transversus
- internal oblique
- external oblique.

They do not end at the sternum, they end at the rectus muscle.

# 5.4 Spleen

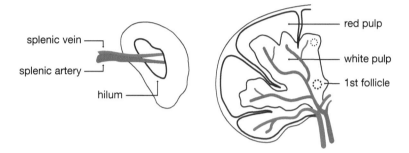

To remember key facts about the spleen use the 1, 3, 5, 7, 9, 11 rule:

It is 1 × 3 × 5 inches in size; it is 7 oz in weight; it is positioned between T9 and T11.

(I know that we use metric units in the UK but for the rule to work we need to have it in imperial figures: 7 oz is approximately 200 g!)

## ARTERIAL AND VENOUS SUPPLY

The arterial supply is from the splenic artery. This is the biggest branch of the coeliac trunk. It passes through the splenorenal ligament and gives off branches to the pancreas and stomach.

The venous drainage is from the splenic vein. It joins the superior mesenteric vein to form the portal vein.

## NERVE SUPPLY

Sympathetic fibres from the coeliac plexus.

## COMPONENTS

There are 4 components:

- Supporting tissue – fibroelastic and forms the capsule.
- White pulp – lymphatic nodules arranged around an arteriole.
- Red pulp – comprises connective tissue and many sinuses filled with blood, hence the red colour. The red pulp contains many cells including lymphocytes, red blood cells and macrophages.
- Vascular system.

This can be remembered using the mnemonic "SHIP":

- **S**torage of red blood cells (8% of circulating RBCs are here).

- **H**aematopoiesis, especially during fetal life and also disease (e.g. CML/myelosclerosis).

- **I**mmune – antigenic stimulation which leads to the formation of plasma cells and increased lymphopoiesis.

- **P**hagocytosis – removes debris and old red blood cells and microorganisms. It is like a 'filter'. It also initiates the humoral and cellular immune response.

# 5.5 Liver

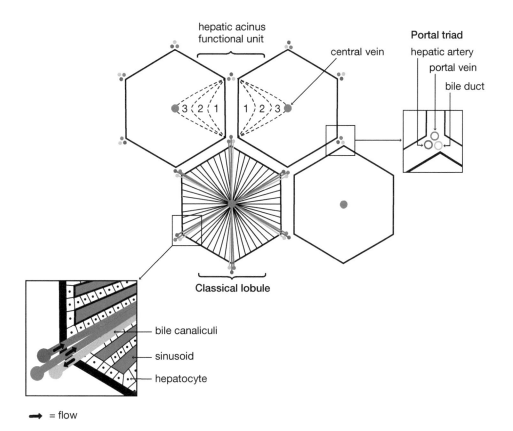

hepatic acinus
functional unit

central vein

**Portal triad**

hepatic artery

portal vein

bile duct

3  2  1    1  2  3

**Classical lobule**

bile canaliculi

sinusoid

hepatocyte

➡ = flow

The liver comes up as a question in the OSCE. You should know the basic anatomy of the portal triad and some facts about blood flow. I will answer some of the questions here.

- The liver is the second largest organ in the body. It weighs approximately 1.5 kg, and receives 25% of blood flow (approximately 1.5 L/min).

- Blood is supplied by the hepatic artery (25%) and the hepatic portal vein (75%); each supply 50% of oxygen.

- Venous drainage is via the left, right and middle hepatic veins to the inferior vena cava (IVC).

- The liver is divided into the right and left lobe by the falciform ligament.

- Functionally, the liver is divided into lobules. Blood enters the lobule through the portal vein and hepatic artery. Blood then flows through sinusoids, lined with hepatocytes, to the central hepatic venule.

- The hepatic acinus is the metabolic unit of the liver. Each acinus comprises a diamond shape that runs between the central veins of two lobules. Within the acinus are hepatocytes; the amount of oxygen that the hepatocytes receive is related to distance from the arterioles. There are 3 zones: zone 1 is best oxygenated (it is nearest the arteriole; see image), whereas zone 3 has the least oxygen and hence is at most risk of ischaemia. Because of this the hepatocytes in zone 1 are specialised for oxidative liver functions (gluconeogenesis), and they are at most risk of blood-borne toxins and deposition of haemosiderin in haemochromatosis. Zone 3 hepatocytes carry out glycolysis, lipogenesis and cytochrome P450 drug detoxification. Hence zone 3 cells are at most risk from $N$-acetyl-$p$-benzoquinone imine (NAPQI) production in paracetamol overdose.

# 5.6 Nephron

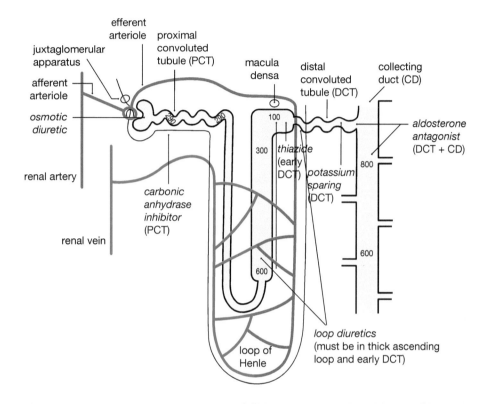

The kidney is a complicated organ which performs many functions.

- It regulates extracellular fluid volume and electrolyte composition, total body water volume, acid–base balance and blood pressure.

- It produces the active form of vitamin D, renin, erythropoietin and glucose and it excretes waste products.

Most people have 2 kidneys. They are located in the upper abdomen in the retroperitoneal space. They are normally approximately 12 cm in length and 150 g in weight. Each kidney has 2 distinct regions: the outer cortex and the inner medulla.

The basic functional unit of the kidney is called the nephron (see figure). There are about 1.5 million nephrons in each kidney! The glomerulus (a capillary network), Bowman capsule, the proximal convoluted tubule (PCT) and the distal convoluted tubule (DCT) are situated in the cortex. The loop of Henle and collecting duct are in the medulla. The PCT reabsorbs electrolytes and water lost from the plasma through filtration at the glomerulus. The loop of Henle descends from the renal cortex into the medulla and then returns to the cortex.

The juxtaglomerular apparatus consists of the macula densa (special cells in the wall of the tubule responsible for sensing and responding to tubular composition) and the afferent arteriole granular cells (cells that secrete renin).

The collecting ducts pass through the renal medulla into the renal pelvis.

Blood supply is via the renal artery, a branch from the abdominal aorta. Venous drainage is via the renal vein into the inferior vena cava (IVC).

Kidneys receive 1 L/min blood flow (20% cardiac output), the cortex receives 90% and the medulla receives 10%. The cortex receives 10 × more blood flow than it needs, for oxygenation, whereas the medulla only just receives enough blood for adequate oxygenation. This is because the flow is needed for filtration (the glomerular filtration rate, GFR).

## Common OSCE question

Describe the different diuretics that work in different parts of the kidney.

- **Osmotic diuretic** (mannitol): inhibits reabsorption of water and $Na^+$, leading to hypertonic hyponatraemia.

- **Carbonic anhydrase inhibitor:** inhibits the enzyme carbonic anhydrase (hydration of carbon dioxide and dehydration of carbonic acid. This causes renal loss of $HCO_3^-$ ion, which carries $Na^+$, $H_2O$ and $K^+$.

- **Loop diuretics:** block $Na^+/K^+/Cl^-$ transporter in the ascending loop of Henle (potassium wasting).

- **Thiazide diuretics:** block $Na^+/K^+$ transporter (potassium wasting).

- **Potassium sparing diuretics** (amiloride/spironolactone): block aldosterone receptors in the cortical collecting duct. This decreases $Na^+$ and water reabsorption and decreases $K^+$ secretion (potassium sparing).

**Blood vessels in the arms**

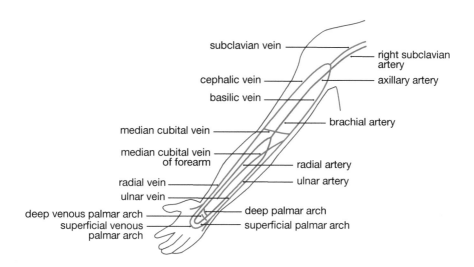

### ARTERIES

- The arteries can be seen as one line from the armpit that forms a loop from the cubital fossa (CF) to the hand.
- The subclavian artery becomes the axillary artery which becomes the brachial artery.
- This then divides in the CF to the radial artery (laterally) and the ulnar artery (medially).
- They join in 2 loops in the hand, the deep palmar arch and the superficial palmar arch.

### VEINS

- The veins start as a shorter line, the subclavian vein, that divides into the cephalic vein (laterally) and the basilic vein (medially).
- These loop from the upper arm down to the hand where it also forms 2 loops, the deep palmar arch and superficial palmar arch.
- The median cubital vein joins the basilic and cephalic veins.
- The median cubital vein drains into the basilic vein.

## 6.2 Brachial plexus

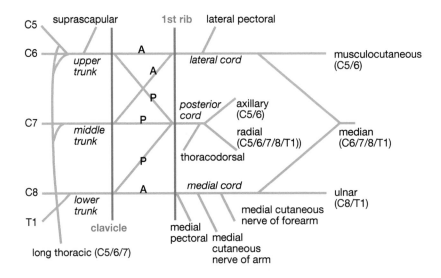

| A | anterior |
| CNA | cutaneous nerve of arm |
| CNF | cutaneous nerve of forearm |
| LT | lower trunk |
| MT | middle trunk |
| P | posterior |
| UT | upper trunk |

## How to draw

### STEP 1

- Draw 3 lines horizontally.
- The middle line should be approximately 2/3 the length of the outside lines.

### STEP 2

- Add in the landmarks: the clavicle and 1st rib. These should be perpendicular lines at approximately 1/3 and 2/3 along the middle line.

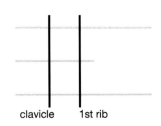

STEP 3

- Add the roots and label: C5, C6, C7, C8 and T1.

- Add in the long thoracic nerve; this usually comes off near the roots of C5, C6 and C7.

- Label the upper, middle and lower trunks.

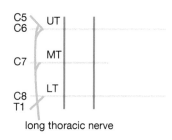

long thoracic nerve

STEP 4

- Draw in the divisions – these usually occur between the clavicle and first rib. Each trunk has an anterior (A) and posterior (P) division.

- Draw them in by drawing an arrowhead from the outer two lines to meet in the posterior cord and then cross the top half of the arrow.

- The posterior division of each trunk joins to form the posterior cord.

- The anterior divisions of the upper and middle trunk join to form the lateral cord and the anterior division of the lower trunk forms the medial cord.

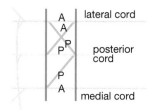

STEP 5

- Draw a second arrowhead joining the lateral and medial cord. These form the median nerve.

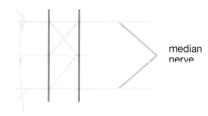

STEP 6

- Draw a 'snake's tongue'; this is the posterior cord dividing to form the axillary nerve (upper) and the radial nerve (lower).

- Label the musculocutaneous (M/C) nerve and the ulnar nerve.

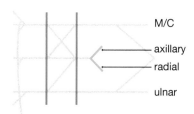

## STEP 7

- Add in one branch from the lateral cord – this is the lateral pectoral nerve.

- Add in three branches from the medial cord – these are the medial cutaneous nerve of the forearm (CNF), the medial cutaneous nerve of the arm (CNA) and the medial pectoral nerve.

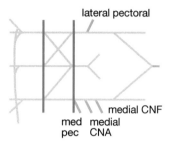

lateral pectoral

medial CNF
med medial
pec CNA

## STEP 8

- Add in one branch from the posterior cord – this is the thoracodorsal nerve (reminder: dorsal and posterior both mean behind/back).

- Add in one branch from the upper trunk – this is the suprascapular nerve (this can be missed in a supraclavicular block; it usually supplies the lateral skin of the shoulder and so can lead to pain in shoulder surgery if missed).

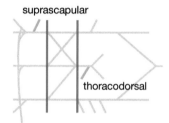

suprascapular

thoracodorsal

# 6.3 Axilla

BB   biceps brachii muscle
BR   brachialis muscle
CB   coracobrachialis muscle
M/C   musculocutaneous nerve

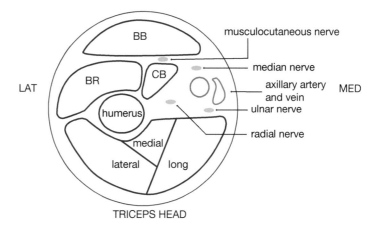

There are few good simplistic versions of the axilla. I found it difficult to represent the anatomy exactly. This diagram should help you label any diagram of the axilla the examiner may show you, but it is not an exact anatomical replica.

## How to draw

### STEP 1

- Draw a large circle to represent the cross-section of the axilla with a small circle in the middle just lateral to the centre – this represents the humerus.

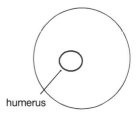

### STEP 2

- Draw a semicircular shape, split into 3, below the humerus. This represents the triceps muscle.

- There are 3 heads: the lateral head (left), the medial head (middle) and the long head (right).

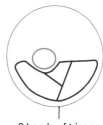

## STEP 3

Draw 3 shapes as shown above the humerus:

- the brachialis muscle
- the biceps brachii muscle
- the coracobrachialis muscle.

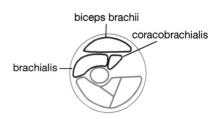

## STEP 4

- Draw a red circle medial to the humerus – this represents the axillary artery.

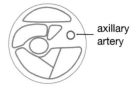

## STEP 5

- Draw a blue shape lateral to the axillary artery – this represents the axillary vein.

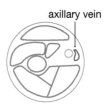

## STEP 6

- Draw 4 green dots, 3 encircling the axillary artery at approximately 12 o'clock (median nerve), 5 o'clock (ulnar nerve) and 8 o'clock (radial nerve), and 1 between the biceps brachii and coracobrachialis muscles, the musculocutaneous nerve (M/C).

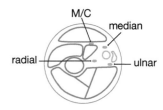

# 6.4 Cubital fossa

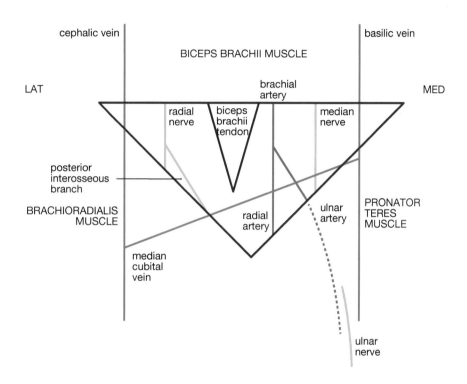

I remember this image by the shape – 'the triangle'. Using different shapes for different areas helps to differentiate them in your mind.

## How to draw

**STEP 1**

- Draw an isosceles triangle pointing downwards. Label the borders: biceps brachii muscle above, pronator teres medially and brachioradialis laterally.

- Draw a smaller triangle just lateral to the centre to represent the biceps brachii tendon.

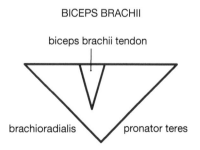

**STEP 2**

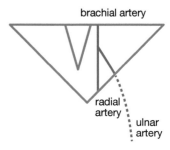

- Draw the brachial artery as a straight line down just medial to the biceps brachii tendon.

- This divides into the ulnar artery medially and the radial artery laterally. The ulnar artery passes under the pronator teres where it joins the ulnar nerve.

**STEP 3**

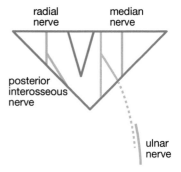

- Add in the ulnar nerve part-way down by the dotted ulnar artery.

- Add in the median nerve medial to the brachial artery.

- Add in the radial nerve lateral to the biceps brachii tendon; draw in the posterior interosseous branch. (This is important because a radial nerve block that is too low can miss this branch and hence the patient can experience wrist pain during surgery.)

**STEP 4**

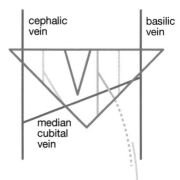

- Add in the veins. Draw an H shape with a diagonal crossbar from lower to higher, lateral to medial.

- Label these: cephalic, basilic and median cubital veins.

**TIP!**

Put your arm out with your thumb pointing upwards. The basilic vein is on the 'base' of the arm and the cephalic vein is nearer the head.

# 6.5 Wrist

FCR  flexor carpi
     radialis tendon
FCU  flexor carpi
     ulnaris tendon
MN   median nerve
PL   palmaris longus
R    radius
RA   radial artery
U    ulna
UA   ulnar artery
UN   ulnar nerve

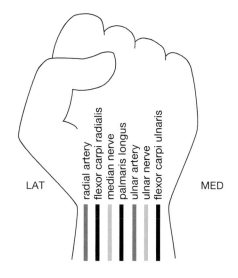

LAT

radial artery
flexor carpi radialis
median nerve
palmaris longus
ulnar artery
ulnar nerve
flexor carpi ulnaris

MED

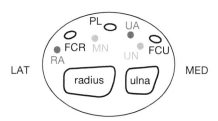

PL  UA

FCR  MN  UN  FCU

RA

LAT

radius  ulna

MED

The wrist is often overlooked for revision of anatomy. However, we commonly put in arterial lines and sometimes perform nerve blocks on the arm and so it is vital we know what lies where. To help remember it, think about the '7 lines' of the wrist.

## How to draw

### STEP 1

- Draw a hand shape.

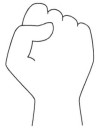

## STEP 2

- Draw 7 lines in the following order: red, black, green, black, red, green and black. The lines represent the tendons (black), nerves (green) and arteries (red).

- From lateral to medial these are: the radial artery, flexor carpi radialis (FCR), the median nerve, palmaris longus, ulnar artery, ulnar nerve and flexor carpi ulnaris (FCU).

- Nerves are often 'protected' by tendons and so you can see that the median nerve lies between and below 2 tendons and the ulnar nerve lies just below FCU.

- The radial artery can be easily found by feeling for FCR and palpating just laterally.

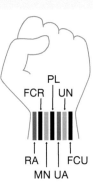

## How to draw the cross-section

### STEP 1

- Draw an oval shape with 2 squares in it to represent the radius and ulna.

### STEP 2

- Draw 7 coloured dots/circles that correspond to the picture above. Note that nerves are deep compared with the tendons.

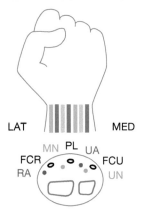

# 7.1 Blood vessels in the legs

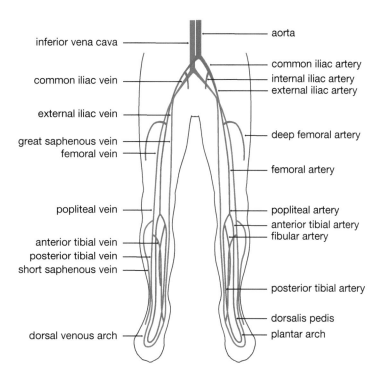

inferior vena cava

aorta

common iliac vein

common iliac artery
internal iliac artery
external iliac artery

external iliac vein

great saphenous vein
femoral vein

deep femoral artery

femoral artery

popliteal vein

popliteal artery
anterior tibial artery
fibular artery

anterior tibial vein
posterior tibial vein
short saphenous vein

posterior tibial artery

dorsal venous arch

dorsalis pedis
plantar arch

This is more complicated than the arm. I have included the main branches of arteries and veins.

### ARTERIES

You can learn the upper half of this diagram in *Section 5.1: Abdominal aorta*.

- The external iliac artery becomes the common femoral artery behind the inguinal ligament.

- The common femoral artery gives off a branch of the deep femoral artery and continues into the thigh to become the superficial femoral artery.

- The superficial femoral artery becomes the popliteal artery.

- It then divides into the anterior tibial artery (becomes the dorsalis pedis artery) and the posterior tibial artery; these join in the foot to form the plantar arch.

- The peroneal artery is a branch of the posterior tibial artery.

**VEINS**

The veins are more complicated.

- The veins start in the foot as a dorsal venous arch; this drains into the posterior tibial vein, the anterior vein and the great saphenous vein.

- The posterior and anterior tibial veins drain into the popliteal vein.

- The popliteal vein becomes the femoral vein; the great saphenous vein drains into the femoral vein.

- The femoral vein becomes the external iliac vein and then this becomes the common iliac vein.

- The common iliac veins join to form the IVC.

# 7.2 Lumbosacral plexus

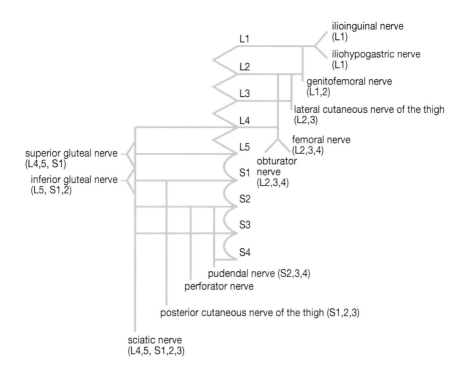

## How to draw

### STEP 1

- Draw 4 arrowheads pointing left and 4 semicircles pointing left below the arrowheads; label the nerve roots as shown.

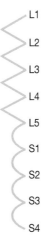

## STEP 2

- Add in the sciatic nerve.

- This has roots L4, 5 and S1, 2 and 3; join them together to form the sciatic nerve.

- Add in the superior gluteal nerve between roots L4, L5 and S1 and the inferior gluteal nerve between roots L5, S1 and S2.

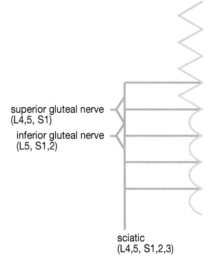

superior gluteal nerve (L4,5, S1)

inferior gluteal nerve (L5, S1,2)

sciatic (L4,5, S1,2,3)

## STEP 3

Add in 3 lines:

- One from S1, 2 and 3 – this is the posterior cutaneous nerve.

- One from roots S2 and 3 – this is the perforator nerve.

- One from S2, 3 and 4 should join to make the pudendal nerve.

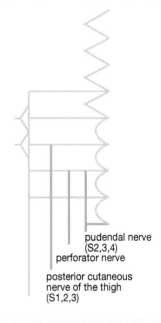

pudendal nerve (S2,3,4)

perforator nerve

posterior cutaneous nerve of the thigh (S1,2,3)

**STEP 4**

Add the lumbar part of the lumbosacral plexus.

- Add one line from L1 which splits into two: the ilioinguinal nerve and the iliohypogastric nerve.

- Add a second line from L2 and join it to L1, to form the genitofemoral nerve.

- Add another line from L3 and join this to L2, to form the lateral cutaneous nerve of the thigh.

- Draw another line from L4, join it to L2 and 3, split it in two and these will be the obturator nerve and femoral nerve.

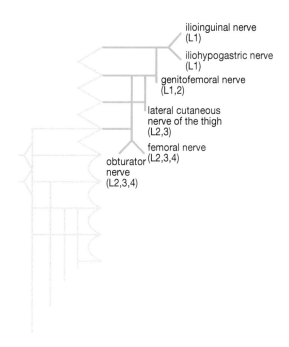

ilioinguinal nerve (L1)

iliohypogastric nerve (L1)

genitofemoral nerve (L1,2)

lateral cutaneous nerve of the thigh (L2,3)

femoral nerve (L2,3,4)

obturator nerve (L2,3,4)

# 7.3 ▶ Femoral canal

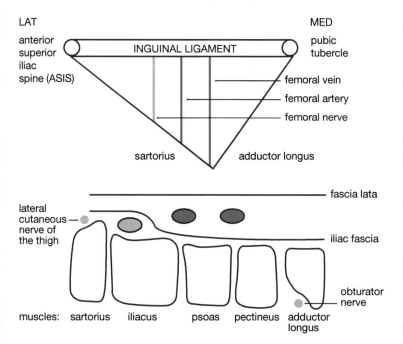

The two images look at the right femoral canal in a schematic way from the coronal view and sagittal view. Some people remember the order of the nerve, artery and vein using the word NAVY, where Y is for Y front!!

## How to draw the coronal cross-section

### STEP 1

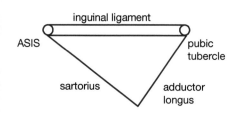

- Draw a down-facing triangle under a horizontal rectangle with two circles at the ends to represent the inguinal ligament.

- The medial end is the pubic tubercle, the lateral end is the anterior superior iliac spine (ASIS).

- The borders below are, medially, the adductor longus muscle and, laterally, the sartorius muscle.

### STEP 2

- Draw a blue line on the medial side from the inguinal ligament to the lower border. This represents the femoral vein.

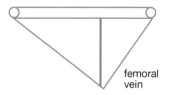

femoral vein

### STEP 3

- Draw a red line down from the middle of the inguinal ligament. This represents the femoral artery.

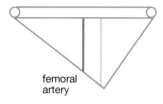

femoral artery

### STEP 4

- Draw a green line on the lateral side from the inguinal ligament to the lower border. This represents the femoral nerve.

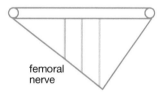

femoral nerve

## How to draw the sagittal cross-section

### STEP 1

- Draw one horizontal line from left to right. Draw a second one below this, narrow at the lateral side and then wider at the medial side (as shown).

- The upper line is the fascia lata and the lower line is the iliac fascia.

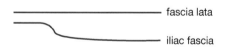

fascia lata

iliac fascia

### STEP 2

- Draw 5 square (ish) shapes below these two lines, as shown. These represent the muscles that lie under/around the femoral triangle.

- The muscles can be remembered with the word 'SIPsPA'; not a real word, but it helped me! From lateral to medial: **s**artorius, **i**liacus, **ps**oas, **p**ectineus and **a**dductor longus.

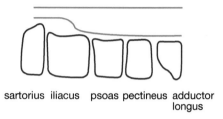

sartorius  iliacus    psoas pectineus adductor
longus

### STEP 3

- With a green pen add in the lateral cutaneous nerve of the thigh, lateral and superior to the sartorius muscle.

- Draw the femoral nerve superior to the iliacus.

- Draw the obturator nerve just below and lateral to the adductor longus muscle.

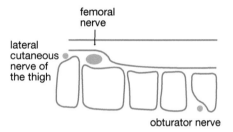

femoral
nerve

lateral
cutaneous
nerve of
the thigh

obturator nerve

### STEP 4

- Draw in the femoral artery and the femoral vein (medially), between the fascia lata and iliac fascia.

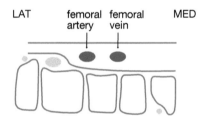

LAT          femoral  femoral        MED
artery    vein

# 7.4 Popliteal fossa

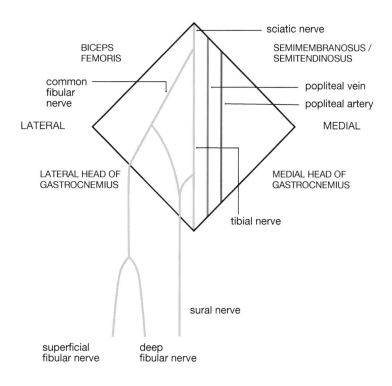

This can be remembered as 'the diamond'.

## How to draw

### STEP 1

- Draw a diamond shape as shown.
- Label the borders: superiolateral is biceps femoris, superiomedial is semimembranosus and semitendinosus, inferolateral is lateral head of gastrocnemius and inferomedial is the medial head of gastrocnemius.

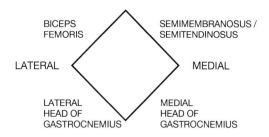

### STEP 2

- Draw a straight red line down, off centre, to represent the popliteal artery (continuation of the femoral artery). The popliteal artery is the deepest structure in this image – an important aspect that may not necessarily be appreciated with a simple 2D drawing.

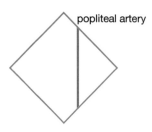

### STEP 3

- Draw a straight blue line lateral to the popliteal artery to represent the popliteal vein. Although they are drawn next to each other, the vein is normally more superficial. The artery is deep to the vein and the nerves are often superficial to both.

- Draw a green line down from upper point to lower point. The top part is the sciatic nerve. This continues distally to become the tibial nerve medially and the common fibular nerve that runs laterally.

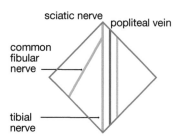

### STEP 4

- Draw in the sural nerve. This can be formed from both the tibial nerve and the common fibular nerve.

- Add in the superficial and deep fibular nerves.

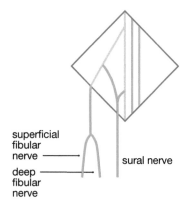

# 7.5 ► Ankle

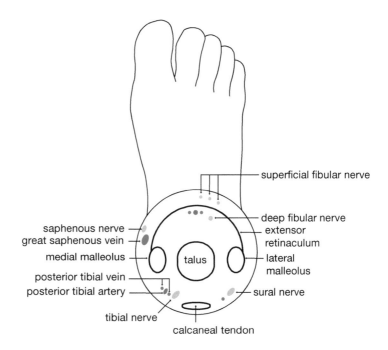

This diagram indicates where the 5 nerves to the ankle are and shows a cross-section from the heel to the forefoot.

I always think it looks like a person wearing headphones and use this to help remind me which diagram it is.

## How to draw

### STEP 1

- Draw a large circle with a smaller circle in the middle – this central circle is the talus bone.

- Draw an oval on both sides of the talus and join them with a semicircular line – these are the malleoli joined by the extensor retinaculum.

- Draw an oval at the base of the circle to represent the calcaneal tendon (or Achilles tendon).

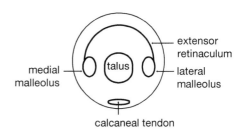

## STEP 2

- Draw a blue dot and a green dot anterior to the medial malleolus – these represent the great saphenous vein (blue dot) and the saphenous nerve (green dot).

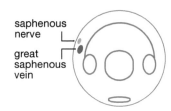

## STEP 3

- Above the extensor retinaculum draw a few green dots to represent the superficial peroneal nerves.

- Below the extensor retinaculum draw one red dot (dorsalis pedis artery), with 2 blue dots (dorsalis pedis veins) and a green dot (deep fibular nerve) laterally.

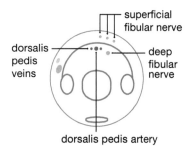

## STEP 4

- Draw the sural nerve (green dot) and the small saphenous vein (blue dot) just posterior to the lateral malleolus and anterior to the calcaneal tendon.

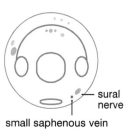

## STEP 5

- Draw the posterior tibial artery (red dot), posterior tibial vein (blue dot) and tibial nerve (green dot), just posterior to the medial malleolus and anterior to the calcaneal tendon. Note that the tibial nerve is sometimes referred to as the posterior tibial nerve; however, this is not the correct name (possibly an error because the tibial vein and artery nearby have posterior as part of their names).

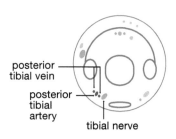

## STEP 6

- Remember that the saphenous nerve is a branch of the femoral nerve, but the other 4 nerves are branches of the sciatic nerve (see *Section 7.4: Popliteal fossa*).

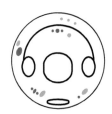